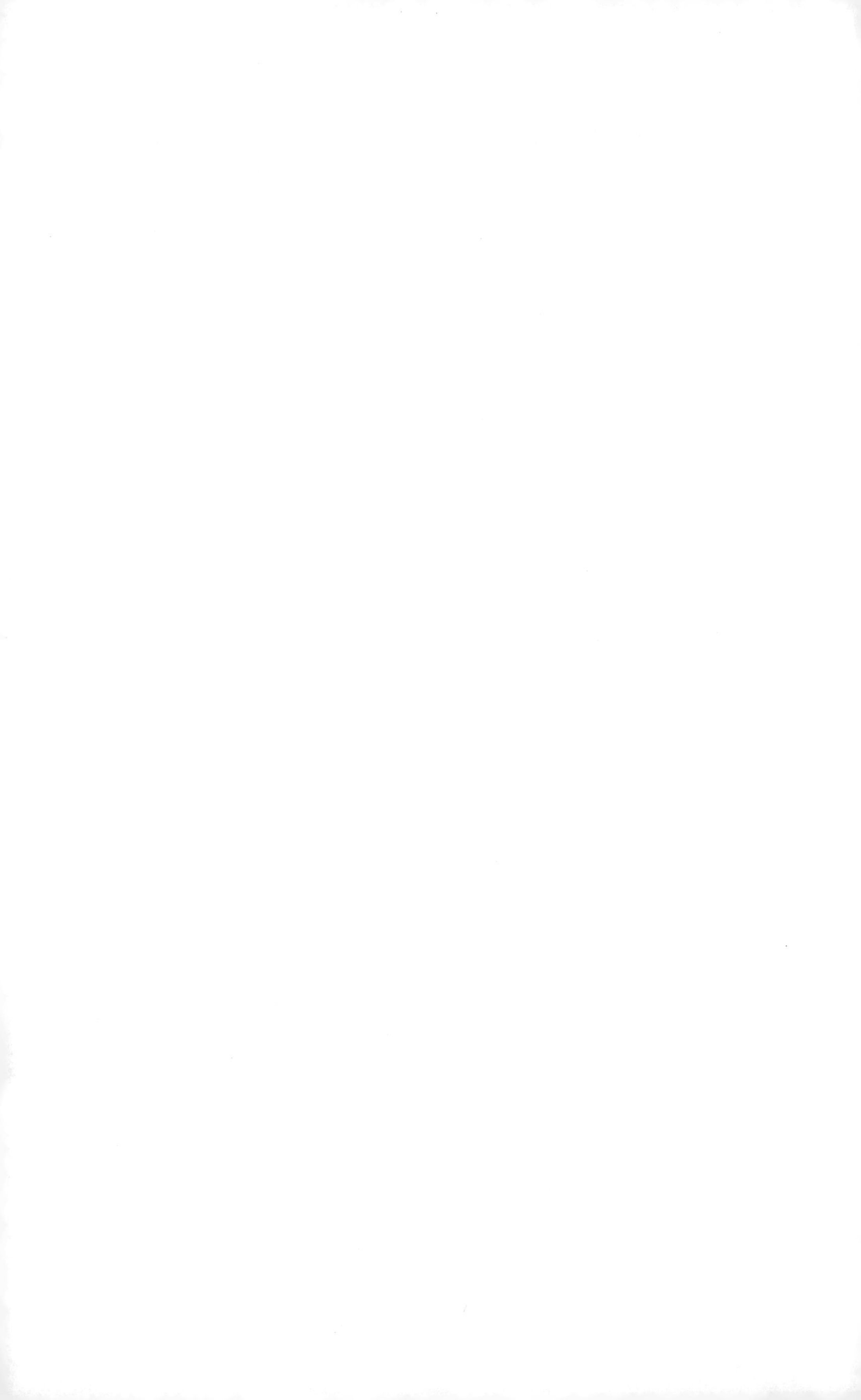

Disruptive Trends in Computer Aided Diagnosis

Chapman & Hall/CRC Computational Intelligence and Its Applications

Series Editor: Siddhartha Bhattacharyya

Intelligent Copyright Protection for Images
Subhrajit Sinha Roy, Abhishek Basu, Avik Chattopadhyay

Emerging Trends in Disruptive Technology Management for Sustainable Development
Rik Das, Mahua Banerjee, Sourav De

Computational Intelligence for Human Action Recognition
Sourav De, Paramartha Dutta

Disruptive Trends in Computer Aided Diagnosis
Rik Das, Sudarshan Nandy, Siddhartha Bhattacharyya

For more information about this series please visit: www.crcpress.com/Chapman—HallCRC-Computational-Intelligence-and-Its-Applications/book-series/CIAFOCUS

Disruptive Trends in Computer Aided Diagnosis

Edited by

Rik Das, Sudarshan Nandy
and Siddhartha Bhattacharyya

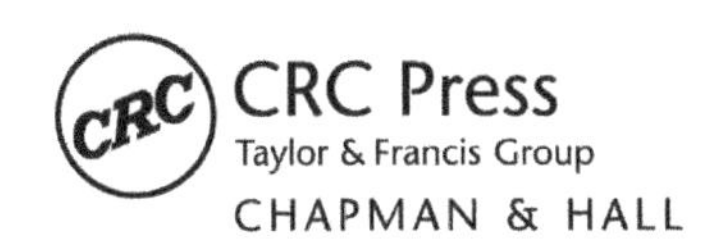

First edition published 2022
by CRC Press
6000 Broken Sound Parkway NW, Suite 300, Boca Raton, FL 33487-2742

and by CRC Press
2 Park Square, Milton Park, Abingdon, Oxon OX14 4RN

Library of Congress Cataloging-in-Publication Data
Names: Das, Rik, 1978– editor. | Nandy, Sudarshan, editor. | Bhattacharyya, Siddhartha, 1975– editor.
Title: Disruptive trends in computer aided diagnosis/edited by Rik Das, Post Graduate Programme in Information Technology, Xavier Institute of Social Service, Ranchi, Jharkhand, India, Sudarshan Nandy, Dept. of Computer Science and Engineering, Amity School of Engineering and Technology, Amity University of Kolkata, Kolkata, West Bengal, India, Siddhartha Bhattacharyya, Department of Computer Science and Engineering, Christ University, Bangalore, Karnataka, India.
Description: First edition. | Boca Raton: Chapman & Hall/CRC Press, 2021. |
Series: Computational intelligence and its applications |
Includes bibliographical references and index. |
Summary: "This book is an attempt to collate novel techniques and methodologies in the domain of content-based image classification and deep learning/machine learning techniques to design efficient computer aided diagnosis architecture. It is aimed to highlight new challenges and probable solutions"– Provided by publisher.
Identifiers: LCCN 2021012293 (print) | LCCN 2021012294 (ebook) |
ISBN 9780367493370 (hardback) | ISBN 9780367493400 (paperback) |
ISBN 9781003045816 (ebook)
Subjects: LCSH: Diagnosis–Decision making–Data processing. |
Clinical medicine–Decision making–Data processing.
Classification: LCC R723.5 .D57 2021(print) |
LCC R723.5(ebook) | DDC 616.07/5–dc23
LC record available at https://lccn.loc.gov/2021012293
LC ebook record available at https://lccn.loc.gov/2021012294

ISBN: 978-0-367-49337-0 (hbk)
ISBN: 978-0-367-49340-0 (pbk)
ISBN: 978-1-003-04581-6 (ebk)

Typeset in Palatino
by Newgen Publishing UK

Rik Das would like to dedicate this book to his father, Mr. Kamal Kumar Das, his mother Mrs. Malabika Das, his better half Mrs. Simi Das and his kids Sohan and Dikshan.

Sudarshan Nandy would like to dedicate this book to his father, Mr. Sukumar Nandy, his mother, Mrs. Anjana Nandy, his loving wife, Mrs. Surabhi Nandy and his son, Samarjit.

Siddhartha Bhattacharyya would like to dedicate this book to Dr. Aparna Chakraborty, Joint Director of Public Instruction, Higer Education Department, Government of West Bengal, West Bengal, India.

Contents

Figures

Tables

Editor Biographies

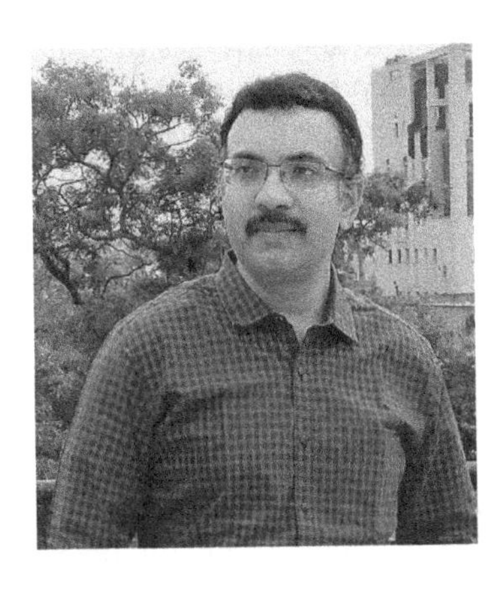

Rik Das is assistant professor for the Post Graduate Programme in Information Technology, Xavier Institute of Social Service, Ranchi, India. He is a PhD (Tech.) in Information Technology from University of Calcutta and received his M.Tech. (Information Technology) from the University of Calcutta after his BE (Information Technology) from the University of Burdwan, West Bengal.

Dr. Das has over 16 years of experience in academia and research with various leading universities and institutes in India, including Narsee Monjee Institute of Management Studies (Deemed-to-be-University), Globsyn Business School, and Maulana Abul Kalam Azad University of Technology. He had an early career stint in business development and project marketing with industries such as Great Eastern Impex and Zenith Computers.

Dr. Das was appointed a Distinguished Speaker for the Association of Computing Machinery, New York, in July, 2020. He is featured in uLektz Wall of Fame as one of the Top 50 Tech Savvy Academicians in Higher Education across India for the year 2019. He is also a member of the International Advisory Committee of AI-Forum, UK.

Dr. Das was awarded with Professional Membership of the Association of Computing Machinery, New York, for 2020–2021. He is the recipient of the prestigious InSc Research Excellence Award hosted in the year 2020. Dr. Das was conferred the Best Researcher Award at the International Scientist Awards on Engineering, Science and Medicine for the year 2021.

Dr. Das has carried out collaborative research with professionals from industries such as Philips-Canada, and Cognizant Technology Solutions. His keen interest in application of machine learning and deep learning techniques for designing computer aided diagnosis systems has resulted in joint publications of research articles with professors and researchers from various universities abroad, including the College of Medicine, University of Saskatchewan, Canada; Faculty of Electrical Engineering and Computer Science, VSB Technical University of Ostrava, Ostrava, Czech Republic; and Cairo University, Giza, Egypt. Dr. Das has filed and published two Indian patents consecutively during the year 2018 and 2019 and has contributed to over 40 international publications to date. He has also authored three books in the domain of content-based image classification and has edited three volumes to date with IGI Global, CRC Press, and De Gruyter. Dr. Das has chaired several sessions in international conferences on artificial intelligence and machine learning as a domain expert.

Dr. Das has been an invited speaker for various national and international technical events, conclaves, meetups and refresher courses on data analytics, artificial intelligence, machine learning, deep learning, image processing and e-learning, organized and hosted by prominent bodies such as University Grants Commission (Human Resource Development Centre), the Confederation of Indian Industry (CII), Software Consulting Organizations, the MHRD initiative under Pandit Madan Mohan Malviya National Mission on Teachers and Teaching, IEEE Student Chapters, and the computer science/information technology departments of leading universities.

Dr. Das has a YouTube channel named "Curious Neuron" as his hobby to disseminate free knowledge and information to larger communities in the domain of machine learning, research and development and open-source programming languages. Dr. Das is always open to discussing new research and project ideas for collaborative work and for techno-managerial consultancies.

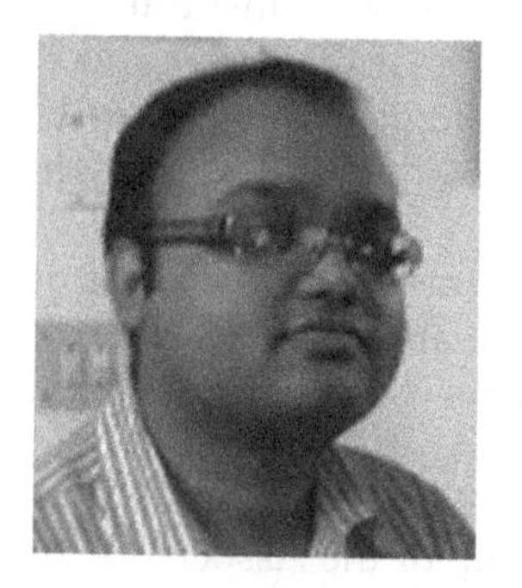

Sudarshan Nandy earned a PhD in Engineering and Technology from Kalyani University, West Bengal, in 2014. Dr. Nandy obtained his M.Tech in Computer Science and Engineering from West Bengal University of Technology in 2007 and his BE degree in Computer Science and Engineering from BPUT, Orissa, in 2004. He is presently assistant professor at the Department of Computer Science and Engineering, Amity School of Engineering and Technology, Amity University. Kolkata. His area of research includes artificial neural network, metaheuristic algorithms, optimization, functional analysis, and cloud computing. He has contributed to many research articles in various journals and conferences and is a member of various professional societies.

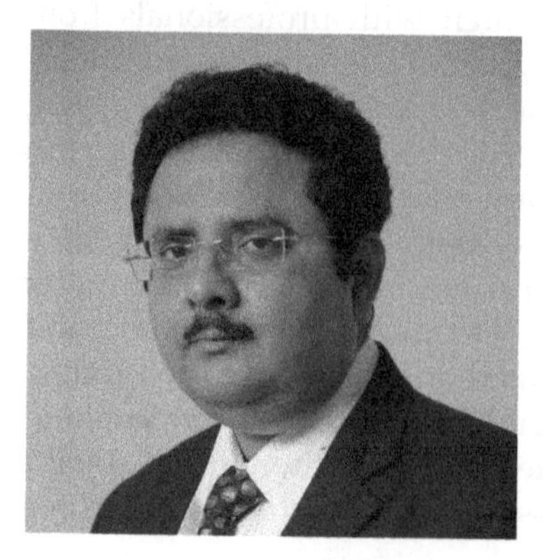

Siddhartha Bhattacharyya received his Bachelors in Physics, Bachelors in Optics and Optoelectronics and Masters in Optics and Optoelectronics from the University of Calcutta in 1995, 1998 and 2000 respectively. He received his PhD in Computer Science and Engineering from Jadavpur University, in 2008. He is the recipient of the University Gold Medal from the University of Calcutta for his Masters. He is recipient of several coveted awards, including the Distinguished HoD Award and Distinguished Professor Award conferred by the Computer Society of India, Mumbai Chapter, in 2017, the Honorary Doctorate Award (D. Litt.) from the University of South America and the South East Asian Regional Computing Confederation International Digital Award ICT Educator of the Year in 2017. He was appointed as the Association for Computing Machinery (ACM) Distinguished Speaker for the tenure 2018–2020 and was inducted into the People of ACM hall of fame by ACM, USA, in 2020. He is the IEEE Computer Society Distinguished Visitor for the tenure 2021–2023. He has been elected as the full Foreign Member of The Russian Academy of Natural Sciences, Moscow, Russia.

Dr. Bhattacharyya is currently the principal of Rajnagar Mahavidyalaya, Birbhum, India. He was a professor in the Department of Computer Science and Engineering of Christ University, Bangalore during December 2019 to February 2021. He served as principal of the RCC Institute of Information Technology, Kolkata, during 2017–2019. He has also served as a Senior Research Scientist in the Faculty of Electrical Engineering and Computer Science of VSB Technical University of Ostrava, Czech Republic (2018–2019). Prior to this, he was the Professor of Information Technology of RCC Institute of Information Technology, Kolkata. He served as the head of the department from March 2014 to December 2016. Prior to this, he was an associate professor of Information Technology of the RCC Institute of Information Technology, Kolkata, from 2011 to 2014. Before that, he served as an assistant professor in Computer Science and Information Technology at the University Institute of Technology, University of Burdwan, West Bengal, 2005–2011. He was a lecturer in Information Technology at Kalyani Government Engineering College, West Bengal, India during 2001–2005. He is co-author of 6 books and the co-editor of 75 books and has more than 300 research publications in international journals and conference proceedings to his credit. He has two PCTs and has been a member of organizing and technical program committees of several national and international conferences. He is the founding chair of ICCICN 2014; ICRCICN, 2015, 2016, 2017, 2018; and ISSIP, 2017, 2018, Kolkata. He was the general chair of several international conferences, such as WCNSSP, Chiang Mai, Thailand, 2016; ICACCP, Sikkim, 2017, 2019; ICICC, New Delhi, 2018; and ICICC, Ostrava, Czech Republic, 2019.

Dr. Bhattacharyya is associate editor of several journals, including *Applied Soft Computing*, *IEEE Access*, *Evolutionary Intelligence* and *IET Quantum Communications*. He is editor of the *International Journal of Pattern Recognition Research* and the founding editor in chief of the *International Journal of Hybrid Intelligence, Inderscience*. He has guest edited for several international journals. His research interests include hybrid intelligence, pattern recognition, multimedia data processing, social networks and quantum computing.

Dr. Bhattacharyya is a life fellow of the Optical Society of India (OSI); life fellow of the International Society of Research and Development (ISRD), UK; a fellow of the Institution of Engineering and Technology (IET), UK; a fellow of the Institute of Electronics and Telecommunication Engineers (IETE), India; and a fellow of the Institution of Engineers (IEI), India. He is also a senior member of the Institute of Electrical and Electronics Engineers (IEEE), USA; the International Institute of Engineering and Technology (IETI), Hong Kong; and the ACM, USA. He is a life member of the Cryptology Research Society of India (CRSI), the Computer Society of India (CSI), the Indian Society for Technical Education (ISTE), the Indian Unit for Pattern Recognition and Artificial Intelligence (IUPRAI), the Center for Education Growth and Research (CEGR), the Integrated Chambers of Commerce and Industry (ICCI), and the Association of Leaders and Industries (ALI). He is a member of the Institution of Engineering and Technology (IET), UK; the International Rough Set Society; the International Association for Engineers (IAENG), Hong Kong; the Computer Science Teachers Association (CSTA), USA; the International Association of Academicians, Scholars, Scientists and Engineers (IAASSE), USA; the Institute of Doctors Engineers and Scientists (IDES), India; the International Society of Service Innovation Professionals (ISSIP); and the Society of Digital Information and Wireless Communications (SDIWC). He is also a certified Chartered Engineer of the Institution of Engineers (IEI), India. He is on the board of directors of the International Institute of Engineering and Technology (IETI), Hong Kong.

Contributors

Md Aziz Ahmad
MECON Limited, Ranchi, India

Siddhartha Bhattacharyya
Rajnagar Mahavidyalaya,
Birbhum, India

Rik Das
Xavier Institute of Social Service,
Ranchi, India

Sourav De
Cooch Behar Government
Engineering College, Cooch
Behar, India

K. D. Desai
Maharshi Parashuram College
of engineering, Mumbai
University, India

Satish R. Devane
University of Mumbai, India

Manjusha Joshi
MPSTME / NMIMS Deemed
University, India

Arana Kausar
Xavier Institute of Social Service,
Ranchi, India

Palash Kumar Kundu
Jadavpur University, India

Pankaj Kumar Manjhi
VinobaBhave University,
Hazaribag, India

Khushbu Kumari
Yogoda Satsanga Mahavidyalaya,
Ranchi, India

Simran Kumari
Amity University, Kolkata,

Madhusree Kundu
National Institute of Technology
Rourkela, India

M. S. Menon
Fortis- S. L. Raheja Hospital,
Mumbai, India

Tamoghna Mukherjee
Amity University, Kolkata, India

Satya Narayan Singh
Xavier Institute of Social Service,
Ranchi, India

Sudarshan Nandy
Amity University, Kolkata, India

Nusrat Parveen
University of Mumbai, India

Anamika Singh
Savitribai Phule Pune University,
Pune, India

Chandrani Singh
Lincoln University Malaysia,
Pune, India

Harish Verlekar
MPSTME / NMIMS Deemed
University, India

Akshay Vinayak
Amity University, Kolkata, India
Kolkata

Preface

Rik Das, Sudarshan Nandy, and Siddhartha Bhattacharyya

Computer Aided Diagnosis (CAD) is an active area of research instrumental for identifying fatal disease at its inception. CAD has achieved noteworthy advancements in this domain with the popularity of current disruptive trends in machine learning applications. A high level of precision superior to manual detection is observed with application of CAD systems in recognizing malignancy for the terminal disease cancer, which has challenged the medical science for an extensive period. This has prevented premature death of many patients due to late detection and several procedural formalities. Therefore, it is pertinent to design efficient algorithms for proposing CAD systems to mitigate the challenges of critical illnesses at an early stage. Researchers are facing multiple challenges for preparing an automated detection system due to lack of training data, sample annotation, region of interest identification, proper segmentation and so on.

Fortunately, recent advancements in computer vision and content-based image classification have paved the way for assorted techniques to address the aforesaid challenges and have helped to attain novel paradigms for designing CAD systems. Popular deep learning and machine learning application have profusely added to augmenting detection accuracy.

The present volume is an attempt to collate novel techniques and methodologies in the domain of content based image classification and deep learning/machine learning techniques to design efficient computer aided diagnosis architecture. It is aimed to highlight new challenges and probable solutions in the domain of computer aided diagnosis to leverage balancing of a sustainable ecology.

The volume comprises ten well-versed chapters on CAD and applications.

Computer aided diagnosis has exhibited immense potential as a research domain in analyzing significant ailments with precision comparable to that of experienced medical practitioners. Advances in medical imaging have further boosted the efficiency of the process in extending its services to the masses. Recently many advancements in the domain of computer aided diagnosis have been observed due to progress in artificial intelligence and machine learning based approaches in assisting medical science. Nevertheless, there are challenges, which include collection of reliable data as one of the important aspects in advancement of CAD. Progress in designing advanced image-capturing devices and efficient segmentation techniques is gradually providing usable insights to deal with the limitations. Chapter 1 discusses the significance of computer aided diagnosis in contemporary times and the future scope for its diversified applications.

Chapter 2 focuses on the relevance of computer aided diagnosis to maintain a sustainable world by providing a detailed review and analysis of the technological aspects. It also discusses the collaborative effect of machine learning in playing a significant role enabling computer aided detection and diagnosis to find a wider and longer trajectory leading to smart healthcare. It also throws light on the long-term negative consequences.

Sustainability is the keyword for growth, be it economic, business or environmental. All nations continuously aspire to grow in various aspects, focusing on a better quality of life for their people. This good quality of life implies happy people blessed with long and healthy lives. Untimely death or living with acute sickness and miseries signifies underdevelopment. Control over epidemics and early detection and cure of deadly diseases is the need of the hour, and CAD can be of great help in winning over life-threatening diseases. Chapter 3 presents the various application areas where CAD can be put to use for the betterment of patients and the society at large.

Generative Adversarial Networks (GAN) advocate sophisticated domain-specific data augmentation by making use of a number of GAN techniques, wherein the accuracy of the results derived from synthesizing, effectually reduces the problem of data scarcity in medical imaging. GANs generally use a generator and a discriminator model that are trained together, in which there is a reproduction of new image and subsequent identification of the original from the generated ones. To optimize on clinical detection and decisions, GANs are used in conjunction with several deep learning models, where the adversarial learnings are used to train them to improve accuracy of segmentation. Chapter 4 presents some of these frameworks, which can then be generalized for CAD(x) or CAD(e). GAN's capability to model high-dimensional data, handling missing data, and making provision for multiple plausible answers in the segment of image synthesis, and translation has culminated in frequent usage of this technique in computer aided diagnosis.

Handling and combatting the alarming spread of Corona Virus Disease 2019 (COVID-19) is the prime concern of global authorities in recent times. Detection and diagnosis of this disease is a major challenge for medical and health personnel due to lack of previous knowledge in dealing this novel outbreak. Researchers are attempting to deploy highly efficient machine learning and deep learning techniques for effective identification of COVID-19. The traditional radiological X-ray, CT scanning and magnetic resonance imaging (MRI) techniques are coupled with an intelligence-based learning system for a preferential outcome to leverage efficient dealing with the detection and diagnosis of the COVID cases with better monitoring approaches. Chapter 5 reviews recent machine learning and deep learning based approaches for detection of corona virus disease. The authors have endeavored to bring assorted propositions under one roof to assist researchers comparing efficiencies of diverse ML techniques for COVID-19 detection. It will create more opportunities for better analyzing and understanding the machine learning and deep based approaches for dealing with COVID-19 and similar unknown threats in times to come.

Heart Rate Variability (HRV) analysis is an authentic tool for cardiac risk stratification and validates the HRV parameters with echocardiogram analysis. The HRV indices derived from Electrocardiograph (ECG) were acquired for 3–5 minutes of diseases population. Statistical independence is ensured by the t-test. Heart rate, Standard Deviation of NN intervals (SDNN), and High Frequency (HF) power are the candidate features. Chapter 6 presents a method for cardiac health assessment using ANN in a diabetic population. The classifier uses the Error Back Propagation algorithm with Artificial Neural Network (ANN). Cluster analysis (k-NN) is based on HRV parameters. Classifier accuracy is 85 percent for 47 epochs with 30 hidden layer neurons. Mean square error (MSE) is 0.000001 at 41st epoch. False positive error is 0 percent and false negative error is 85.4 percent. The results of the cluster analysis are validated with Left Ventricular Ejection Fraction (LVEF). Four clusters are identified based upon the quantitative analysis of feature sets, based on the risk. Validation of the maximum cluster is cross-checked by the LVEF.

Early diagnosis and expedited medical intervention are critical factors in reducing mortality rates associated with Myocardial Infarction (MI). Machine Learning (ML) programs perform better with experience. In Chapter 7, experiences and information of expertise are used. Dissemination of knowledge to answer queries along with study of numerous algorithmic programs that improved mechanically through expertise were done, and this was possible through ML. The information of algorithm that may offer the most effective result to classify knowledge as MI or MI not, Support Vector Machine (SVM) that performs well compared with alternative ML algorithm like Naïve Bayes (NB), Logistic Regression (LR), Decision Tree (DT), Random Forest (RF) and so forth were worked with. The model accuracy depends on the datasets available, and the features used to predict the model. If SVM doesn't give better accuracy than other models such as ensemble algorithm, neural network too can be applied to get better diagnosis from the model.

Chapter 8 proposes a photoplethysmography (PPG) based non-invasive, rapid, inexpensive, automated diagnostic and decision support tool for cardiovascular ailments. An indigenous, cost effective setup consisting of microcontroller based data acquisition with computerized signal processing and diagnostic software is presented in an entrepreneurial spirit. The PPG signature was obtained using infrared light through the fingertip in reflectance mode. A study on accumulated PPG signatures with 15 volunteers (pertaining to age group ranging from 11–12 years, 21–25 years, 35–40 years and 50–62 years) was carried out. The fiducial points of PPG and its first- as well as second-degree derivative (SDPPG) waveforms are used to obtain valuable information on untimely arterial stiffness, and cardiovascular health in general. The developed indigenous system consists of (i) PPG waveform acquisition system. (ii) data pre-processing, (iii) PPG beat extraction, (iv) analysis of the extracted PPG waveform to identify fiducial points, and (v) estimation of clinical parameters including photoplethysmographic augmentation index (PPGAI), instantaneous heart rate, variability of heart rate in time domain and point care plots offering information about non-linear HRV. The proposed automated device was developed and implemented in the MATLAB Environment.

The COVID-19 disease that originated from the SARS-CoV-2 virus is spreading exponentially among the populated countries. In India, the spread of the virus and the number of people infected are increasing every day. In this scenario, administration has imposed lock-down procedures to break the chain of virus spread. This measure reduces the chances of infection as the person in good health can avoid coming into contact with infected persons. Society, however, cannot afford the lock-down process for an unknown period of time because economic and social activity are also halted. In this situation, the spreading behaviors of virus in various communities constitute essential information to administrations.

The best procedure to acquire that information is to analyze a different forecasting model for the epidemic, a model that provides prediction of infected and recovering cases from this viral disease. In Chapter 9, the spreading behavior of COVID-19 epidemic is analyzed by means of comparing the ARIMA prediction model for infected and recovered cases. Epidemic models are tested over the data reported by the health ministry of different states in India. The study of this chapter is performed over Delhi, West Bengal, Tamilnadu, and Maharashtra. The statistical analysis based model selection process proves the efficacy of the selected model.

Finally, Chapter 10 concludes the volume with directions for the future and of research and innovation perspectives computer aided diagnosis and allied fields.

This volume would come to the benefit of a wide range of professionals including medical practitioners, medical researchers, bachelors and masters students of computer science, virology, electronics and information science. The editors would find it rewarding if the present volume comes to the use of mankind and society.

1

Evolution of Computer Aided Diagnosis: The Inception and Progress

Rik Das, Siddhartha Bhattacharyya, and Sudarshan Nandy

CONTENTS

1.1 Introduction

Computer aided diagnosis (CAD) has secured enormous relevance as one of the most significant research arenas in the medical and health sectors due to its advanced and real-time usefulness in detection and diagnosis of medical cases [1]. CAD can be prominently categorized into two distinct segments, namely, computer aided detection (focuses on discovering the medical diseases) and computer aided diagnosis (instrumental in diagnosing diseases and prescribing medication remedies). The traditional computer aided diagnosis was attempted for the first time at the era of 1960s [2]. Since then, CAD rapidly emerged with its vast applications in the field of medical diagnosis during the 1980s, and now it has become the most significant approach for detection and diagnosis of medical diseases, with the increasing popularity of deep learning and other advanced automated techniques. Traditional CAD has higher dependencies on physicians and the medical team for monitoring the medical cases [3]. But the scenario for automated CAD has experienced a paradigm shift from the traditional system. At present, CAD is not only useful for detection and diagnosis of medical diseases without human assistance, but also it is applied for regulating the medical cases with minimum involvement of medical team restricted to scoring better performance accuracy [4]. This minimizes the performance time as well as improves the work productivity. Computer aided diagnosis, based on various advanced automated techniques such as Convolutional Neural Network (CNN), deep learning methods, and traditional machine-learning techniques, has delivered better precision in diagnosing ailments when compared to seasoned physicians. Advanced techniques for content-based image processing for robust descriptor definition has made CAD a major tool to analyze radiological images like computed tomography (CT) scanning, X-rays of various body parts and MRI (magnetic resonance imaging) scans, and so forth. The image shown in Figure 1.1(a) is a mammogram that is further processed using image binarization to create Figure 1.1(b). The image shown in Figure 1.1(b) has clearly segregated the foreground and background and has highlighted the object of interest for further analysis.

Therefore, the multidimensional contribution of computer aided diagnosis has effectively boosted the confidence of medical practitioners to trust in a second opinion that has high precision. The arrangement has saved many lives and proven to be beneficial in determining a line of treatment for faster recovery.

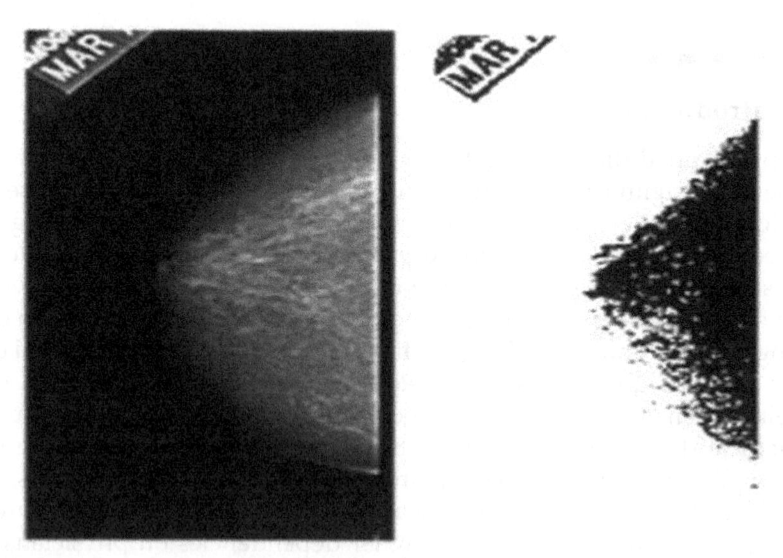

FIGURE 1.1
Binarization of Mammogram.

1.2 Literature Survey

The contribution and importance of computer aided diagnosis for medical applications cannot be overlooked in the contemporary period [5]. It is recognized as an important tool for monitoring medical cases in the fields of public health and medication [6]. CAD has not only contributed to detecting and diagnosing diseases but is also used for monitoring or regulating the workload of clinical teams with higher performance accuracy. In the field of medical imaging computer aided diagnosis is used as an active agent to analyze and yield resourceful insights about the disease from the information stored in the image and is otherwise not being comprehended by manual investigation. Computer aided diagnosis has been contributing since 1960s in the field of medical science with its diverse automated applications [7]. Figure 1.2 shows a chronological journey of computer aided diagnosis [8].

Some drawbacks of the traditional CAD – such as equal participation of medical team, more processing time and unclassified databases and so forth – have been overcome with the automated CAD, which have associated with real-time results with less processing time and more accurate performance [9] [10].

The second era of CAD started in the mid-1980s to the 1990s and has come up with new technologies such as artificial intelligence and other techniques [11]. The novel technologies have immensely aided better performance in medical diagnosis with the help of high-resolution images, quick-decision support approaches and other optimizational techniques for reading and understanding medical data proficiently [12].

A CAD system based on artificial intelligence techniques is proposed to diagnose neurological disorder in the human brain with the help of various feature extraction methods [13].

FCN (fully convolutional network) along with bidirectional long- and short-term memory (LSTM) are designed for breast cancer diagnosis [14]. A deep-learning based computer aided diagnosis system has recorded valuable results in diagnosing diabetic retinopathy that detects and divides segments and classifies the images of Diabetic Retinopathy for achieving better performance in terms of accuracy [15].

A research-proposed ensemble model of CAD with diverse classifiers named k-nearest neighbors (KNN), probabilistic neural network (PNN), neural network (NN), support vector machine (SVM), and so forth. The work has achieved significant improvements in results for diagnosis of medical cases through radiological images of the liver system [16].

A novel proposition named COVIDiag has been designed for diagnosing COVID-19 cases with the help of CT scan images of corona-virus-infected and non-infected patients [17].

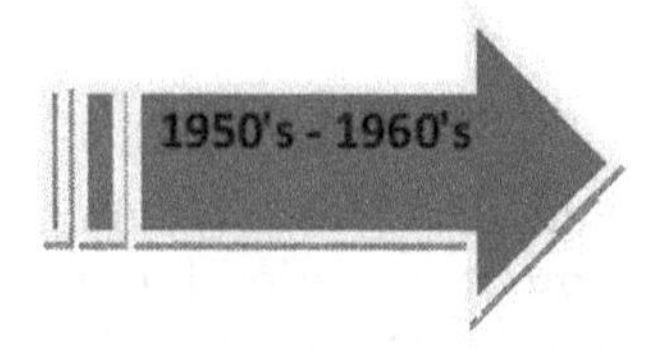

- At its inception it was referred as "Expert Systems in Medicine" [10].
- Further research initiated attempts on developing fully automated "expert systems"

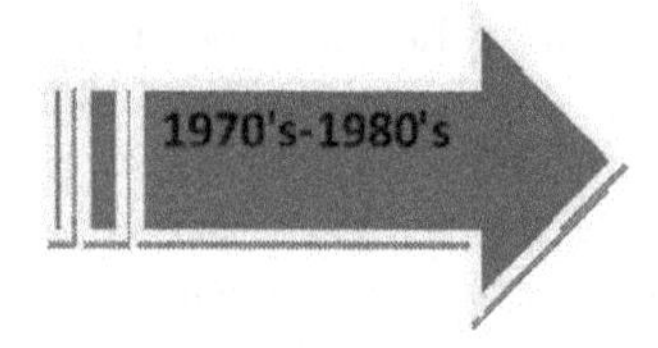

- Karp's discovery on solving complex computational problems by addressing algorithmic complexity limitations [11]
- Now CAD system are considered more as diagnosing aiding tools
- The rule based expert system MYCIN [12]
- Multiple and Complex diagnosis with the Experimental Computer Program INTERNIST-I [13]
- The expert system named CADUCEUS [14]

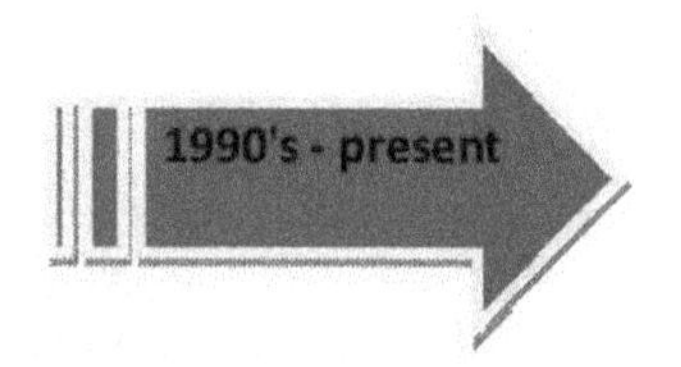

- Landmark approval by FDA for the first CAD system in 1998 (for mammography screening mammography)[15]
- Development of diverse CAD applications in mammography, dealing with dementia and lung diseases[16]

FIGURE 1.2
Chronological Journey of Computer Aided Diagnosis.

In the field of medical diagnosis CAD is contributing continuously with results, and also there has been a lot to do improving the consequences, with much accuracy and less processing time. Thus, it demands more and more research, in the concerned domain, to lead a better medical and health system around the world.

1.3 Data Preprocessing Illustration for Computer Aided Diagnosis

Computer aided diagnosis is successfully implemented in diagnosing severe disorders, including melanoma, breast cancer, diabetes retinopathy and so on [18] [19] [20]. The usefulness of CAD systems has been immensely highlighted in the current COVID 19 pandemic to provide insights for drug discovery to save the human race.

An example of data preparation for the CAD system is shown in Figure 1.3. The image shown in Figure 1.3(a) is of melanoma, a deadly variant of skin cancer. A ground tooth image is shown in Figure 1.3(b). The two images, Figure 1.3(a) and 1.3(b), are multiplied to each other to generate the image in Figure 1.3(c), which is highlighting only the areas of interest. The unwanted regions of Figure 2(a) are not visible in Figure 1.3(c). This kind of morphological operation is indeed helpful in designing input data with portions of images having maximum contribution to the descriptor definition for CAD systems.

The basic image processing shown in Figure 1.2 results in higher accuracy in automated disease detection using CAD compared to traditional methods involving time-consuming and inaccurate manual intervention.

1.4 Future Scope

Computer aided diagnosis is defined as the intersection of medical science and computer science, as illustrated in Figure 1.4. It facilitates interdisciplinary exchange of knowledge and ideas among researchers in these two domains and helps in addressing some critical challenges and threats in medical analysis.

Nevertheless, the future scope of CAD will depend on addressing effectively the challenges in the domain, which involves collection of data, appropriate techniques for medical image segmentation, advanced methodologies for descriptor definition, improved data mining and classification techniques for higher precision, efficiently handling big data, strategizing performance assessment standardization for CAD systems and practicing adoption of the CAD system in the clinical process.

The widespread applications of machine-learning and deep-learning techniques are to a great extent handling the challenges of data categorization and image segmentation, and with enhanced accuracy. Advanced imaging techniques and ready availability of high-end imaging devices are assisting tremendously in data collection for development of CAD. Determining the

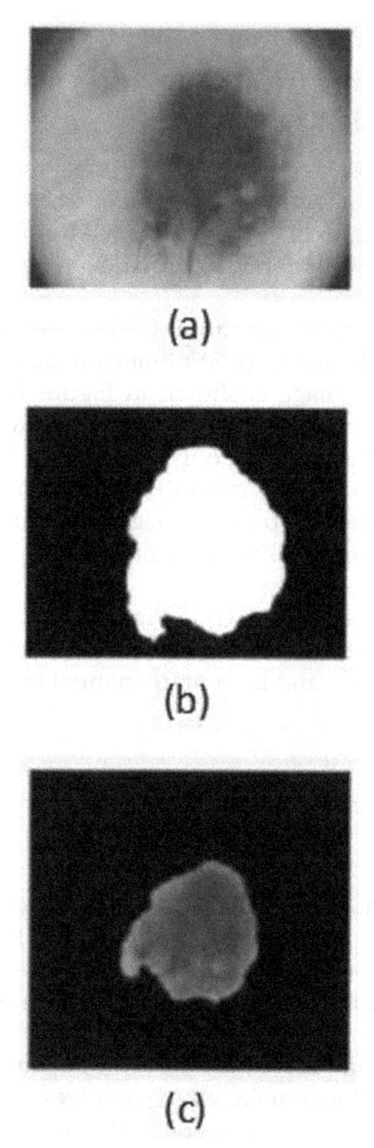

FIGURE 1.3
Identifying Region of Interest.

line of treatment for colonoscopy has been efficiently carried out by using computer aided polyp detection. Schizophrenia patients are diagnosed using a bi-objective technique for CAD. Chest radiography has become very popular and is a reliable means of data sources to enable diagnosis. Moreover, breakthrough results are achieved in detecting potentially lethal disease such

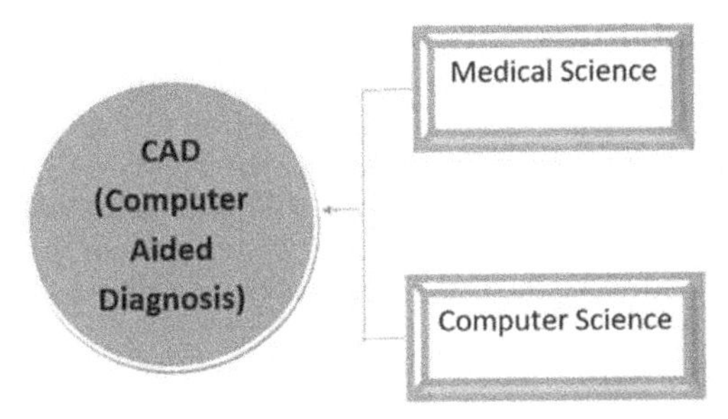

FIGURE 1.4
Computer Aided Diagnosis as a Collaboration of Medical Science and Computer Science.

as cancer with the help of computer aided diagnosis, which is opening up advanced treatment methodologies for faster cures.

Therefore, advancement in either field will lead to a mutual progress of CAD-based assistance towards building a sustainable society.

1.5 Conclusion

Computer aided diagnosis is counted as one of the significant approaches in the field of medical diagnostics. It has leveraged new avenues to early detection and treatment of critical ailments. Computer aided diagnosis helps in faster detection by minimizing the wait time for the arrival of a domain specialist to identify a particular disease. This is usually made possible with the help of the latest advancements in the domain of machine learning and artificial intelligence. With its wide-ranging, effective applications in detection and monitoring of diseases, computer aided diagnosis has become a trusted companion of many medical practitioners. In the near future, computer aided diagnosis will be used as an effective alternative to minimize the clinical workload for the management of medical cases and will be instrumental in setting up a foundation for the public health sector with its many assorted applications.

References

1. Giger, M.L., & Suzuki, K. (2008) Computer-aided diagnosis. In *Biomedical information technology* (pp. 359–374). Academic Press.

2. Loh, B., & Then, P. (2017). Deep learning for cardiac computer-aided diagnosis: benefits, issues & solutions. *mHealth* 3(45), 1–10.
3. Morales, J.M., Ruiz-Rabelo, J.F., Diaz-Piedra, C., & Di Stasi, L.L. (2019) Detecting mental workload in surgical teams using a wearable single-channel electroencephalographic device. *Journal of Surgical Education*, 76(4), 1107–1115.
4. Yanase, J., & Triantaphyllou, E. (2019) A systematic survey of computer-aided diagnosis in medicine: Past and present developments. *Expert Systems with Applications*, 138, 112821.
5. Doi, K. (2007) Computer-aided diagnosis in medical imaging: Historical review, current status and future potential. *Computerized Medical Imaging and Graphics*, 31(4–5), 198–211.
6. Das, R., De, S., Bhattacharyya, S., Platos, J., Snasel, V., & Hassanien, A.E. (2019, March) Data augmentation and feature fusion for melanoma detection with content based image classification. In International Conference on Advanced Machine Learning Technologies and Applications (pp. 712–721). Springer, Cham.
7. Wardle, A., & Wardle, L. (1978) Computer aided diagnosis–a review of research. *Methods of Information in Medicine*, 17(01), 15–28.
8. Bakkouri, I., & Afdel, K. (2020, June) DermoNet: A computer-aided diagnosis system for dermoscopic disease recognition. In International Conference on Image and Signal Processing (pp. 170–177). Springer, Cham.
9. El-Baz, A. et al., (2013) Computer-aided diagnosis systems for lung cancer: challenges and methodologies. *International Journal of Biomedical Imaging*, 2013.
10. Doi, K. (2005) Current status and future potential of computer-aided diagnosis in medical imaging. *The British Journal of Radiology*, 78(suppl_1), s3–s19.
11. Ganguly, A., Das, R., & Setua, S.K. (2020, July) Histopathological image and lymphoma image classification using customized deep learning models and different optimization algorithms. In 2020 11th International Conference on Computing, Communication and Networking Technologies (ICCCNT) (pp. 1–7). IEEE.
12. Raghavendra, U., Acharya, U.R., & Adeli, H. (2019) Artificial intelligence techniques for automated diagnosis of neurological disorders. *European Neurology*, 82(1–3), 41–64.
13. Budak, Ü., Cömert, Z., Rashid, Z.N., Şengür, A., & Çıbuk, M. (2019) Computer-aided diagnosis system combining FCN and Bi-LSTM model for efficient breast cancer detection from histopathological images. *Applied Soft Computing*, 85, 105765.
14. Asiri, N., Hussain, M., Al Adel, F., & Alzaidi, N. (2019) Deep learning based computer-aided diagnosis systems for diabetic retinopathy: A survey. *Artificial Intelligence in Medicine*, 99, 101701.
15. Bansal, S., Chhabra, G., Chandra, B.S., & Virmani, J. (2019) A hybrid CAD system design for liver diseases using clinical and radiological data. In *U-Healthcare Monitoring Systems* (pp. 289–314). Academic Press.
16. Ardakani, A.A., Acharya, U.R., Habibollahi, S., & Mohammadi, A. (2020) COVIDiag: A clinical CAD system to diagnose COVID-19 pneumonia based on CT findings. *European Radiology*, 1–10.
17. Das, R., Ghosh, S., Khatua, S., Sen, A., Thepade, S., & Banerjee, M. (2018, July) Significant bit contribution in Robust Feature Extraction for dermoscopic image

classification. In the 2018 International Conference on Recent Innovations in Electrical, Electronics & Communication Engineering (ICRIEECE) (pp. 2347–2350). IEEE.
18. Shen, L., Margolies, L.R., Rothstein, J.H., Fluder, E., McBride, R., & Sieh, W. (2019) Deep learning to improve breast cancer detection on screening mammography. *Scientific Reports*, 9(1), 1–12.
19. Gargeya, R., & Leng, T. (2017) Automated identification of diabetic retinopathy using deep learning. Ophthalmology, 124(7), 962–969.
20. Thepade, S.D., Jadhav, K., Sange, S., & Das, R. (2020) COVID19 identification from chest x-ray using local binary patterns and multilayer perceptrons. *Journal of Critical Reviews*, 7(19), 4277–4285.

2

Computer Aided Diagnosis for a Sustainable World

Anamika Singh

CONTENTS

2.1 Introduction

2.1.1 Background and Evolution

In the field of medical science, precision and accuracy are most important, as the field is about life-related issues. All decisions of medical practitioners depend upon the health issues detected and diagnosed. Previously, when the diagnosis was based upon symptomatic detection, accuracy was not expected; lately, however, pathological indications have become very helpful. Diseases such as cancer – a major public health issue with very high mortality – requires detection and diagnosis to be done with accuracy. Diagnosis with high accuracy of such disease is only possible when computed and interpreted by computer. Manual diagnosis has many limitations and, thus, needs computer aided detection and diagnosis. It is imperative to have early detection of crucial diseases.

If we dig deeper we may find that application of CAD can be observed back in 1950 (Lusted LB, 1955). A mathematical model of CAD was introduced by Lusted, allowing for the application of CAD to be observed in medicine. Chronologically, in 1963 chest radiograph computer analysis was done. Further, in 1964 Becker's measurement of the cardiothoracic ratio used an automatic method. If we see the analysis done in 1960s we may find that the assumptions during those days were about the replacement of radiologists by computers. The general assumption was made because tasks such as computation/detection can be done better by computers and thus detection of diseases can be improved. This was the time of automated computer diagnosis. In those days the computer was not as powerful as it needed to be to give anticipated results such as advance image processing or access of digital image. Thus, the basic reason was over-expectation from the computer. The computer was to be treated as an aid to decision making, but not to replace the diagnosticians. Thus, it was acknowledged that computers would function as an aid to radiologists not to replace them. Thereafter, the concept of computer aided diagnosis emerged. Initially there was great apprehension about this concept, and the researchers and scientists were skeptical about the CAD schemes. However, all these apprehensions proved wrong.

These apprehensions were based upon the failed attempt of researches in the development toward automated computer diagnosis. However, we see in the present scenario that both automated computer diagnosis and computer aided diagnosis exist. Many scientists believe that in the future the entire CAD scheme will be converted into automated computer diagnosis. There are many common features in CAD and automated computer diagnosis, but many differences also exist. The common factor between computer aided diagnosis and automated computer diagnosis is that they both have analyzed digital medical images, and these have the basis of computer algorithms.

Followed by Ledley in 1966, and in 1973 by Toriwaki, application of CAD for diagnosis was acknowledged. In 1976, Winsberg brought forth a CAD application for mammography. Initially, the development of CAD was gradual, and from the late 1960s until the early 1980s, major development was not evident; however, in 1990s significant development was observed (Wang and Yu, 2019). In the University of Chicago department of radiology, very systematic research had started massively in the 1980s in the Kurt Rossmann Laboratories for Radiologic Image.

The development of computer aided diagnosis started with various schemes. CAD was based upon mathematical and statistical methods and there were theories and models such as Bayes theorem, the maximum likelihood model, and the sequential model, which used to be considered the basis for computer aided diagnosis. For diagnosis and medical processing in the field of computer aided diagnosis, various algorithms and quantitative methods were used to detect and diagnose. Later, in the 1990s, the brilliant evaluation method of "Artificial Neural Network" (ANN) came into the picture, which welcomed the gleaming concept of artificial intelligence. Since artificial intelligence is the intelligence of the machine, unlike natural intelligence, precision in terms of interpretation could have been expected more by now. When intelligence is aided by computer, more precision can be observed. If we analyze the working principle of the artificial neural network (ANN) it works like the human brain and, since it is aided by the machine, the recall rate is very high. This has been proved in various researches. If we see the performance in classification and diagnosis, it is far better and, thus, ANN can be considered as one of the most advanced artificial intelligence technologies (Wang and Yu, 2019). As discussed above, CAD was expected to give a complete diagnosis with the help of machines, which is beyond the capacity, and thus in early 1990s the pace of development was reduced – later, however, development was significant.

In 1993, Wu and associates developed the first computer aided diagnosis model with the help of the Artificial Neural Network, which had the capacity of lesions detection, whether malignant or benign. This study pioneered field of computer aided diagnosis, characterizing abnormality besides the detection or locating of it. During this period the models for making this study were more robust; the models used were the Bayesian Network (BN) and the artificial neural network (ANN) and produced better results. This study proved that it gave better results than diagnosis without computer aid. In 1964 a study by Baker and associates had a more complex model, again based on the artificial neural network. In this study the input data was Breast Imaging and reporting Data System (BI RADS). Further, in 1997, Fogel and associates did the study based on the ANN model, which worked like second opinion to radiologists. Later Kahn and associates came up with Bayesian Network (BN) models that had capability to classify benign and malignant conditions. The Baynesian Network had

TABLE 2.1

Summary of Evolution of Computer Aided Diagnosis Based on Various Models

Study	Year	Objective of Study	Base Model	Ref No.
Lusted LB	1955	Electric phenomena in the human body	Mathematical model	17
Becker et al.	1964	Measurement of cardiothoracic ratio used an automatic method	Digital Image analysis	4
Toriwaki et al.	1973	Acknowledgement of application of CADx for the diagnosis	Graphics & Image processing	22
Winsberg et al.	1967	Detection by means of optical scanning and computer analysis	Optical scanning and computer analysis	25
Wu et al.	1993	First CADx model with ANN	ANN	26
Baker et al.	1995	One of the earliest mammography CADx models built using artificial neural networks	ANN	3
Fogel et al.	1997	Use of ANN examining suspicious masses	ANN	11
Kahn et al.	1997	BN models to classify mammographic lesions as benign and malignant	BN	15
Chhatwal J et al.	2009	CADx model to differentiate between benign and malignant findings	LR, BN & ANN	7

ANN: Artificial Neural Network; LR: Logistic Regression; BN: Bayesian Network

the capacity to help the diagnosticians in their decision making. In later stages, few scientists, such as Chhatwal in 2009 and Burnside in 2010, with a large data set, did the research, and the model used by them were logistic regression (LR) and the Bayesian network (BN) respectively. These scientists used mammography records that gave better results using computer aided diagnostic models than did radiologists. These studies kept on proving that computer aided diagnostic models always gave better results. In 2010, a few scientists such as Ayer, Alagoz, Chhatwal, and Burnside declared that, with the use of artificial neural, the ability of the CADx model to differentiate between benign and malignant, made the findings of this study very significant. Also, it has the ability to analyze the risk: identifying whether it falls in low or high risk. This led to classifying and categorizing the patients and allowed patients to categorize in lower and higher risk groups. This allowed the diagnosticians better risk communication and addresses the patients more efficiently.

2.1.2 Meaning and Significance

"Computer-aided detection" refers to pattern-recognition software that identifies suspicious features on the image and brings them to the attention of the radiologist, in order to decrease false-negative readings (Castellino, 2005). The established computer programs that have been used for medical practice also assist radiologists to find out the prospective abnormalities diagnosed by radiologists. As discussed by Ronald A. Castellino in his article in 2005, "Computer aided detection has been approved by FDA and CE for both screening and diagnostic exams." However, Computer aided diagnosis is different concept from computer aided detection. This defines that when we discuss diagnosis this refers to the analysis of findings in examination. The software in computer aided diagnosis analyses the radiographic findings. Radiographic analysis is done in two stages, that is, in the first stage it is just observed, which means visual perception is done, and in second stage it is analyzed. It can be also explained as a diagnosis in which a computer is used as a tool for generating the result and helps the medical practitioners who make the complete diagnosis. And the end result is based on a computer algorithm.

Also, it can be that detection focuses on localization, and diagnosis emphasizes characterization. That is, computer aided detection will find the area in which cancer occurs, and computer aided diagnosis characterizes the disease as to whether it is in a benign or malignant stage. In other words, the final goal of computer aided diagnosis can be achieved with the help of computer aided detection, which therefore implies that computer aided detection is basis of computer aided diagnosis. To make the clinical diagnosis process medical image processing combines together with computer technology and make the diagnosis more accurate and precise. A flowchart in Figure 2.1 explains the entire process.

The significance of computer aided diagnosis is to have more precision and accuracy. This implies that it increases the rate of disease detection and potential abnormalities and reduces the rate of observational oversight. This becomes the substitute for second observer and reduces the need for well-trained radiologists for observation and analysis. As mentioned above, it allows for making decisions more swiftly for detection and diagnosis. It is different from automated computer diagnosis because it uses computer analysis as a second opinion, and the opinion of computer and physician are considered. In the automated computer diagnosis, the diagnosis is only on the basis of a computer algorithm. In other words it is an assisting tool to the radiologist (Doi, 2007). Thus, it has the potential to improve detection and diagnosis, both. Furthermore, it can be put forth in such a way that CAD has the potential to identify the abnormalities that can elude professionals. The difference between computer aided detection and computer aided diagnosis is that detection highlights the parts that are visibly identifiable, or the structures in the image and the computer aided diagnosis evaluates those

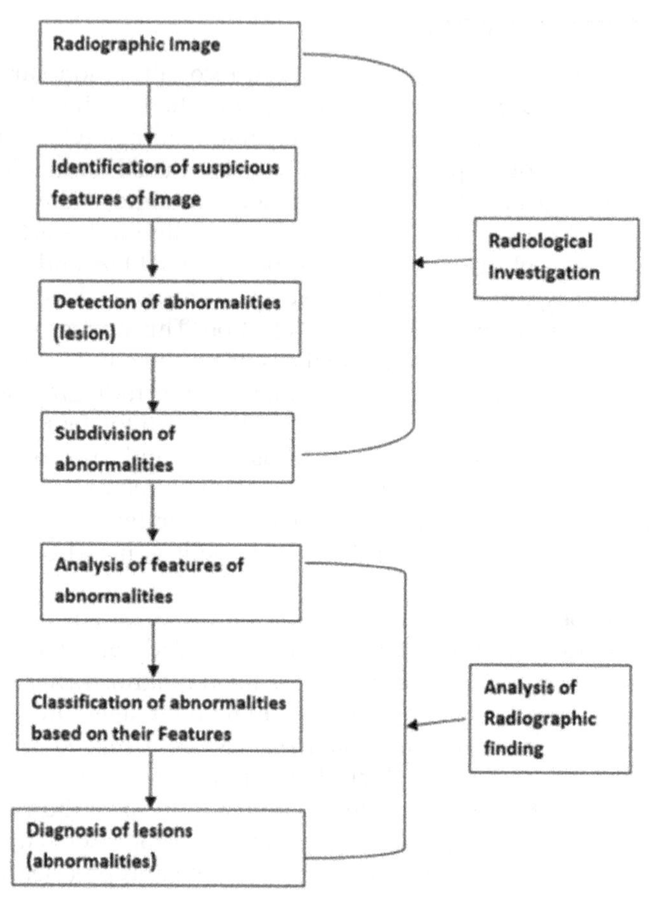

FIGURE 2.1
Flowchart of Computer Aided Diagnosis with Processing Technology of Radiographic Image and Computer.

identified structures (Halalli and Makandar, 2018). It helps the radiologists interpret various medical images such as MRI, ultrasound, x-rays, mammography, and so forth. As mentioned above, it is considered a "second opinion" but it cannot be considered as a substitute for radiologists, and thus it aids the decision-making process. Just by improving the precision of computer aided diagnosis, treatment and cure can be improved. As discussed by Halalli and Makandar, there are few computer aided diagnosis systems that give improved results in terms of detecting the diseases; architectural distortions are the basic challenges. Moreover,Makandar and Halalli have highlighted that the algorithm for computer aided diagnosis will always depend upon accuracy, sensitivity and false identifications. They have indicated in their study that, to design a CAD model, proper technique selection at each stage of medical image analysis is quite important.

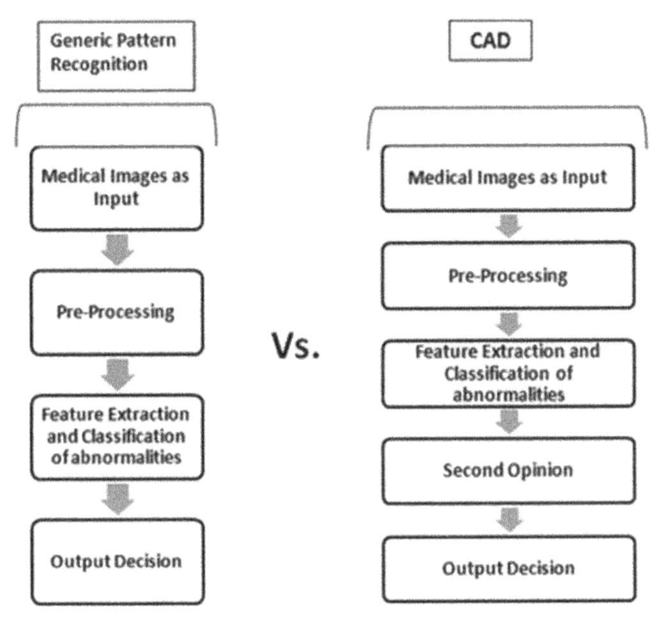

FIGURE 2.2
Difference between General Pattern Recognition System versus CAD.

Thus, the following figure can describe the difference between general pattern recognition and CAD and its significance. This describes and emphasizes how CAD augments the decision of radiologists. CAD aids the decision of radiologists as a second opinion and does not act as an output decision. Hidetaka Arimura (2009), in his study, describes that both systems, that is, the general pattern recognition system and the CAD system comprise pre-processing, feature extraction and classification. Figure 2.2 depicts the difference between the general pattern recognition system and computer aided diagnosis

2.2 Challenges for Computer Aided Diagnosis

Challenges to develop the detection and diagnosis systems are manifold. As we know, to have accurate detection and diagnosis, the proper algorithm is required, and to attain the proper algorithm, segmentation of the data is required. Furthermore, this seeks the trained radiologists who have acumen to evaluate and interpret the results. Besides, there are challenges in developing the design in the computer assistance system and also the implementation of the same offers a challenge. These all are the challenges in the ecosystem of computer aided detection and computer aided diagnosis. Machine learning and deep learning augment the accuracy and precision in detection and diagnosis. Moreover, artificial intelligence (AI), augmented reality (AR), multimodal imaging and so forth aid the computer assisted diagnosis. This has been profoundly supplementing the entire system. The entire ecology of computer aided detection and computer aided diagnosis systems is being augmented by these advancements and assorted techniques. Aforesaid challenges also add the challenge of deployment of these computer assisted techniques and thus the training for those who evaluate the results. These challenges can be overcome by probable solutions that will lead to a sustainable ecology for computer aided systems in the field of medical science. In 2019 Juri Yanase and associates discussed the challenges and, by overcoming those challenges, a sustainable ecology for CAD can be visualized.

The following can be considered as major challenges in the field of the computer aided diagnosis system.

2.2.1 Data Acquisition and Its Assessment

For the computer aided diagnosis, not only good quantities of data but good quality of data are required. Few countries have developed good electronic data for the quality assessments at various hospitals. These records are called electronic health records (EHR). Unfortunately, the recording of data is not done as sincerely as expected. Although the quantity of data is huge, the quality of the data is still in question. To maintain electronic health records, a proper course of action, strategy or guidelines must be followed diligently in order to assure the safety of patients. It is very important for this to have quality assessments, for which there should be credible data that should be assessed with accuracy and precision (Weiskopf and Weng, 2013).

Also, one major challenge in quality of data is the bias. Data are characterized for diseases, but if the sampling of data is not adequately done then chances of bias increase. Thus, to reach a statistically significant result, rich data should be analyzed.

2.2.2 Segmentation of Acquired Data

As we know, the acquired data are processed, and the processing part includes segregation and features identification or extraction. Segmentation is done for large group data such as images. The 2D and 3D images are divided based on their uniformity. Although the algorithm has been developed to segment or divide the data, and these data could be multidimensional, the need of advanced segmentation of data is of utmost importance. Processing of data and the presentation or visualization of data are possible only when advanced segmentation becomes possible. Segmentation is done with various approaches. Some include deep learning techniques to solve the complex problems (Yanase et al, 2019). Since multidimensional images have become very important and bring good results after analysis, advanced techniques for analysis of multidimensional images requires development.

2.2.3 Feature Extraction / Selection

Acquisition of huge data and its segmentation should be followed by feature extraction and feature selection. In feature extraction the relevant data creates a set or subset of features and feature selection, identifying or selecting only relevant information from original data. This can also be explained as feature extraction, which creates new attributes, whereas feature selection keeps a subset of existing attributes (Liu and Motoda, 2012). In feature extraction and selection, deep learning techniques are also included.

This step is very important because huge data are acquired to develop the algorithm. This huge data must be extracted features, as this occupies a large storage space and increases the complexity. Large memory space and computing power are required. The significance of this step is to save space time and memory space, and further helps in the classification step. These steps of developing algorithms for effective feature extraction and selection are very important for the entire computer aided diagnosis system (Newell et al., 2010).

2.2.4 Classification of Data and Data Mining Approaches

Data-mining and machine-learning techniques are used for classification of data. In the entire process of computer aided diagnosis, developing a processing module is very important, and that leads the diagnostic decision. When the dataset is acquired, various classifiers are applied to it to form a cluster. It has been observed that various methods are used, but in a few cases some methods perform phenomenally on some set of data under observation. The reason for this outperformance is not known and, thus, it can be assumed that it differs from case to case. The two methods, supervised learning approaches and unsupervised learning approaches, are usually practiced. Clustering of datasets based on their similarities is the most challenging task. As discussed above, the computer aided diagnosis and the decision taken to diagnose the disease becomes robust when the clustering and classification of data and methods to process it become clear and accurate. Also, misclassification of the data is another big challenge. The cost of a false-positive and a false-negative diagnosis is again a big challenge. Also, over-diagnosis, that is, when a disease or condition is present but in reality poses no significant harm to the patient (Yanase et al., 2019). This has been explained by the example of prostate cancer in old age which, when diagnosed, will not be a big threat but, if notified the patient may have more anxiety and will cause more danger.

2.2.5 Challenge of Big Data

Enormous quantities of data are available, but the processing and analysis of the data is important. The entire quantity of data is not used, only a portion of it. Analysis of this big data, which is defined in three aspects – that is, volume, variety and velocity – is the biggest challenge of computer aided diagnosis (Yanase et al., 2019). The volume of the data can be understood in such ways that even a single test of one patient generates lot of data, and it becomes huge. "Variety" of data can be understood as the data are in various forms, such as semi-structured and unstructured. Human efforts are required to understand and analyze the unstructured data. "Velocity" can be understood as the data to be interpreted in real time; otherwise, the significance of data gets lost. There are several solutions to this big-data analysis and processing, and these solutions such as Apache, Hadoop and Spark are commercially available.

The challenge lies in processing, integrating, analyzing and interpreting in real time. The computer aided analysis system needs to incorporate various approaches with the help of various technologies in order to cater to this challenge.

2.2.6 Standardized Performance Assessment Approaches

It is very important to have standardized performance approaches for computer aided diagnosis. In assessing the effectiveness of computer aided diagnosis there is lack of standard approaches for evaluation (Gallas et al., 2012). In the processing part of computer aided diagnosis – which is done after acquiring the data, that is, pre-processing and main-processing and includes the classification and clustering – misclassification happens. The cost of this misclassification – that is, false-positive or false-negative classification – is high and needs to be addressed. Accuracy in classification is expected and, thus, the significance of a standardized process of assessment for entire computer aided diagnosis is there. Although various methods are discussed that can be applied to assess computer aided diagnostic performance, such as Area Under Curve (AUC), Precision Recall (PR) and so forth, none of these is absolute and covers all aspects of assessment. In order to cover all aspects of the performance of computer aided diagnosis, the Computer Aided Detection in Diagnostic Imaging Subcommittee (CADSC) has been formed for a standardized assessment approach and uses image analysis. The committee has standardized an approach to some extent and also includes other aspects, such as increasing professional awareness and understanding (Petrick et al., 2013). The goal of this committee is not just to establish a standardized creative approach but also to increase professional awareness for CADSC and also understanding the effectiveness and the challenges the committee faces. Other approaches, such as the American Association of Physicists in Medicine

(AAPM), also allow evaluating performance. However, this approach needs tremendous development.

2.2.7 Adoption of Computer Aided Diagnosis in Clinical Practice

Besides mammography, computer aided diagnosis is not practiced very pervasively. The reason for not practicing computer aided diagnosis in a non-mammography system is not having the standardized approach for the performance assessment of computer aided diagnosis (Petrick et al., 2013).

Although various studies have proved the diagnosis system's result to be very encouraging, the validation of algorithms for other medical conditions and other clinical practices has not been done. There are many other fields, such as education and training, where computer aided diagnosis is brought into practice but, as said above, besides mammography, computer aided diagnosis systems is not practiced for other medical conditions. This system is probably limited to mammography because it needs more validation and feedback from clinicians and researchers (Cahan and Cimino, 2017). Another reason can be the training of radiologists and physicians. Many researchers explain it as major reason of poor performance of the CAD system (Regge and Halligan, 2013). There have been other reasons that keep discouraging medical practitioners when it comes to adopting computer aided diagnosis systems in clinical practices. Some contradictions have been highlighted by a few researchers that computer aided diagnosis systems are not as effective and as useful as claimed, and thus insurance companies do not cover claims made for computer aided diagnosis, which further discourages medical practitioners and adoption in clinical practices (Yanase et al., 2019).

2.3 Sustainability

To have a sustainable ecology, the medical field needs to have likely solutions to the challenges facing computer aided systems. The various challenges to acquiring data, processing and utilizing it for decision making with the help of interpretation, need to be addressed. Acquiring the data and dealing with big data with various techniques need accuracy and precision as this data is considered highly sensitive. While classifying and clustering the data, misclassification happens, which projects false-negatives or false-positives. This requires apt training of physicians in order to achieve accurate results. Some researchers and studies have proved the result of absolute(100%) classification results such as the study by Abd-Ellah in 2016. His study has presented the results of presence or absence of brain tumor and its classification into benign or malignant through a computer aided diagnosis system. The CAD system was used for detection and classification. This reached to the accuracy of 100 percent. This proves the potential of computer aided diagnosis for the classification. Overcoming the challenges discussed above and coming out with probable solutions also effectively support that the system needs to be developed in order to develop sustainable ecology for computer aided diagnosis.

Computer aided diagnosis has been among the most sought-after studies for medical researchers. Although this system and the related studies are really complex and tremendous efforts have been made to work on its challenges, yet it is not used in many medical conditions and thus reflects the infrequent clinical use.

It is inevitable that computer aided diagnosis will lead the path of the medical field towards more powerful detection and diagnosis. It is surely going to change the way medicine is practiced. The development of technology has made it possible to have huge data in the medical field, and the analytics for this data has enabled medical practitioners to develop electronic health records, despite having huge data processing and diagnostic errors, which is the hurdle in this field and thus suitable training is expected for processing and visualization. Also, the technology has brought expert medical practitioners across globe on one platform and has allowed them to get connected in real time. This projects the need for a next-generation diagnosis support system (NGDSSs) (Cahan et al., 2017).

2.3.1 Attainment of sustainability

A sustainable ecology for computer aided diagnosis can be developed only when the future of this diagnosis will have an improved version in terms of all the challenges being faced in either algorithmic aspect (this includes developing advanced segmentation approaches; developing advanced feature extraction / selection approaches; developing better classification and other data mining approaches; dealing with big data) or in regulatory aspects (this includes developing standardized performance assessment for CAD Systems and adopting CAD Systems for clinical practice). As we know, development that meets the needs of the present without compromising the ability of future generations to meet their needs is called sustainable development and, if we find the solution by having collaboration between medical practitioners and computer science researchers, a sustainable ecology for the computer can be envisaged in the future. Contribution of developing algorithms wherein improving quality data collection and its assessment can be attained by having good collaboration with computer science researchers and by providing proper training to the physicians' quality assessment can be accomplished. The accuracy of assessment training of medical practitioners becomes very important. Several technologies, such as data mining, machine learning, deep leaning, artificial intelligence, and so forth, are related to computer science, and these technologies assist in developing the algorithm and give promising results. This entire ecology is supposed to develop not only the standardized performance assessment but also a complete feedback system to be provided to the researchers in order to complete the cycle for further improvement in an entire computer aided diagnosis system. As discussed above, this will not only pave the way for the future of a computer aided diagnostic system but also to the other related field of computer science and will take it to the next level practices(Yanase et al., 2019).

2.3.2 New Paradigm

2.3.2.1 Cohorting and Characterizing Disease

Next Generation Diagnosis Support Systems (NGDSS) call for a structured pattern of the patient's presentation by which it is possible to group the patients with similar structured patterns and that would surely give better, dependable and precise results.

2.3.2.2 Full-Cycle Feedback and Training

NGDSS calls for full-cycle feedback that promotes the view of medical practitioners giving feedback to the researchers and ask the clinicians to receive feedback from the patients in order to get more clarity instead of diagnosing on a trial-and-error basis. It also very strongly supports the view about improved training for medical practitioners, which will enable them to interpret the result more accurately.

2.3.2.3 Power of Real Time Clinical Data

Early detection is one of the most important features. Real-time clinical data would enable the clinician in early detection of any disease outbreak. This will allow the clinicians to identify the disease even before the regulatory agency can identify it. This will deter the spread of diseases. This also will enable clinicians to detect groups of patients having the same pattern of disease or having unusual cases in real time, and further will allow taking control measures (Cahan, A. et al., 2017).

2.3.2.4 Better Healthcare in Even Modest Means

Small economies or countries having limited resources can also have improved healthcare in case of NDSS. In most of the published reports of medical researchers, the population living in this setup are not represented to

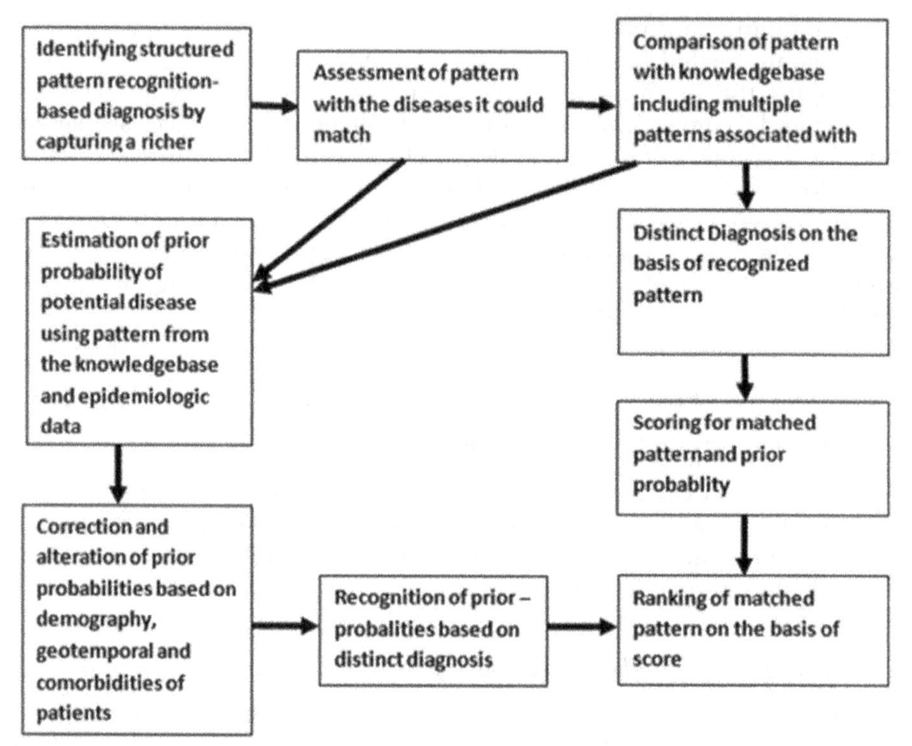

FIGURE 2.3
Conceptual Framework for Next Generation Diagnosis Support System.

a good extent and thus proper healthcare is not possible. In this setting, there are more chances of diagnostic error as there is scarcity of professionals who diagnose and of the test to diagnose it with. Since NGDSS enable professionals to come on one global platform, it will reduce bias by collecting, analyzing and interpreting and also sharing the local knowledge. In the study of Cahan and Cimino, it is clearly portrayed that to have effective next-generation diagnosis systems (NGDSS) the entire framework can be conceptualized in following ways:

(1) Support pattern recognition-based diagnosis by capturing a richer clinical picture;
(2) Provide personalized prior-probability assessments;
(3) Maintain a comprehensive and current knowledge base, and
(4) Better align with clinicians' workflow.

This following picture (Figure 2.3) distinctively depicts the conceptual framework for a next generation diagnosis support system.

2.4 Conclusion

The early development of computer aided diagnosis initially proclaimed it as interference and a burdensome tool. Whereas it was the tool that assisted the radiologists, physicians or diagnostician and later was being considered as something that may even replace the diagnosticians. There was much apprehension about this tool and, therefore, the development of computer aided diagnosis was deferred. Many who were advocating for this tool also had apprehensions and often went back and forth from advocating to being skeptical. Later, into the picture came the discussion for the standardization and calibration of the machines, which was based upon enhancing the performance of entire system (Dolan, 2006).

For a sustainable ecology, computer aided diagnosis needs to be more robust, and the challenges faced by this diagnostic support system need to be overcome. The pattern developed to assist the diagnosis and develop the algorithm need a proper collection of data from the researchers and from its analysis and interpretation. There are several tools to do the same such as data mining, deep learning, machine learning, artificial intelligence, and so forth. To deal with big data some standardized process is expected. As discussed above, various challenges including those discussed in the paper of Juri Yanase, can be overcome, and sustainable development can be expected by evolving the process for an entire ecology and developing the technology.

The framework developed by Cahan and Cimino conceptualizes the NGDSS and discusses improvising the entire ecology. Developing the proper algorithm with the help of technology and appropriate training for the diagnosticians who interpret the data are the key to overcoming the challenges. Also, collaboration between the computer science researchers and medical practitioners will pave the way for a complete feedback cycle which, in turn, will aid the sustainable ecology for computer aided diagnosis. We are aiming at a well-developed computer aided diagnosis system that will change the way medicine is practiced.

References

Arimura, H., Magome, T. et al. (2009) Computer-aided diagnosis systems for brain diseases in magnetic resonance images, *Algorithm*, 2: 925–952. ISSN 1999-4893.

Baker, J., Kornguth, P., Lo, J., Williford, M., & Floyd, C., Jr (1995) Breast cancer: prediction with artificial neural network based on BI-RADS standardized lexicon. *Radiology*, 196(3): 817–822.

Becker, H.C., Nettleton, W.J. Jr, Meyers, P.H., et al. (1964) Digital computer determination of a medical diagnostic index directly from chest X-ray images. *IEEE Transactions on Biomedical Engineering*, 11: 67–72.

Burnside, S., Alagoz, O., et al. (2010) Computer-aided diagnostic models in breast cancer screening. *Imaging in Medicine*, 2(3): 313–323.

Castellino, R.A. (2005) Computer-aided detection (CAD): An overview. *Cancer Imaging*, 5: 17–19. 10.1102/1470-7330.2005.0018 [PMC free article] [PubMed] [CrossRef] [Google Scholar] from: *Computer-aided diagnosis in medical imaging: historical review, current status and future potential.*

Cahan, A. &Cimino, J.J. (2016) A learning health care system using computer-aided diagnosis. *Journal of Medical Internet Research*. 2017 Mar 8; 19(3): e54. doi: 10.2196/jmir.6663. www.jmir.org/2017/3/e54/ [PMC free article] [P u b M e d] [CrossRef] [Google Scholar].

Chhatwal, J., Alagoz, O., Lindstrom, M.J., Kahn, C.E., Shaffer, K.A., & Burnside, E.S. (2009) A logistic regression model based on the national mammography database format to aid breast cancer diagnosis. *American Journal of Roentgenology*, 192(4): 1117–1127.

Doi, K. (Jun-July, 2007) Comput med imaging graph. 31(4–5): 198–211. doi:10.1016/j.compmedimag.2007.02.002. Epub 2007 Mar 8. PMID: 17349778.

Dolan, B. (2006) Computer aided diagnosis in mammography: Its development and early challenges, *Circuits, Systems and Computers*, DOI: 10.1109/ACSSC.2006.354864 Source: IEEE.

Fogel, D.B., Wasson, E.C., Boughton, E.M., Porto, V.W. (1997) A step toward computer-assisted mammography using evolutionary programming and neural networks. *Cancer Lett*, 119(1): 93–97.

Gallas, B.D., Chan, H.P., D'Orsi, C.J., Dodd, L.E., Giger, M.L., Gur, D., Krupinski, E.A., Metz, C.E., Myers, K.J., Obuchowski, N.A. & Sahiner, B. (2012) Evaluating imaging and computer-aided detection and diagnosis devices at the FDA. *Academic Radiology*, 19(4): 463–477.

Halalli, B. and Makandar, A. (2018) Computer aided diagnosis: Medical image analysis techniques. *Breast imaging*, p. 85. http://dx.doi.org/10.5772/intechopen.69792.

Kahn, C.E., Roberts, L.M., Shaffer, K.A., & Haddawy, P. (1997) Construction of a Bayesian network for mammographic diagnosis of breast cancer. *Computers in Biology and Medicine* 27(1): 19–29.

Liu, H. & Motoda, H., (2012) Feature selection for knowledge discovery and data mining. *Springer Science & Business Media* (Vol. 454).

Lusted, L.B. (1955) Medical electronics. *The New England Journal of Medicine*, 252: 580–585.

Makandar, A., & Halalli, B. (2018) Computer aided analysis: Medical image analysis techniques. intechopen69792: 85–109.

Newell, D., Nie, K., Chen, J.H., Hsu, C.C., Hon, J.Y., Nalcioglu, O. & Su, M.Y. (2010) Selection of diagnostic features on breast MRI to differentiate between malignant and benign lesions using computer-aided diagnosis: Differences in lesions presenting as mass and non-mass-like enhancement. *European Radiology*, 20(4): 771–781.

Petrick, N., Sahiner, B., Armato, S.G., Bert, A., Correale, L., Delsanto, S., Freedman, M.T., Fryd, D., Gur, D., Hadjiiski, L. & Huo, Z. (2013) Evaluation of computer-aided detection and diagnosis systems. *Medical Physics*, 40(8).

Regge, D. & Halligan, S. (2013) CAD: How it works, how to use it, performance. *European Journal of Radiology*, 82(8): 1171–1176.

Toriwaki, J., Suenaga, Y., & Negoro, T., et al. (1973). Pattern recognition of chest X-ray images. *Computer Graphics and Image Processing*, 2: 252–271.

Wang, L. & Yu, L. (2019). Computer-aided diagnosis for biomedical applications, computer architecture in industrial, biomechanical and biomedical engineering, IntechOpen, DOI: 10.5772/intechopen.88835. Available from: www.intechopen.com/books/computer-architecture-in-industrial-biomechanical-and-biomedical-engineering/introductory-chapter-computer-aided-diagnosis-for-biomedical-applications.

Weiskopf, N.G. & Weng, C. (2013) Methods and dimensions of electronic health record data quality assessment: enabling reuse for clinical research. *Journal of the American Medical Informatics Association*, 20(1): 144–151.

Winsberg, F., Elkin, M., Macy, J. Jr, et al. (1967) Detection of radiographic abnormalities in mammograms by means of optical scanning and computer analysis. *Radiology*, 89: 211–215.

Wu, Y., Giger M, Doi, K., Vyborny, C., Schmidt, R., & Metz, C. (1993) Artificial neural networks in mammography: application to decision making in the diagnosis of breast cancer. *Radiology*, 187(1): 81–87.

Yanase, J. & Triantaphyllou, E. (2019) The seven key challenges for the future of computer-aided diagnosis in medicine. *International Journal of Medical Informatics*, 129: 413–422.

3

Applications of Computer Aided Diagnosis Techniques for a Sustainable World

Arana Kausar and Aziz Ahmad

CONTENTS

3.1 Introduction

A healthy life is expected of all human beings irrespective of their age or geographic location or economic condition. But for many, this life is never actually experienced. Since time immemorial, there is evidence of different types of diseases being prevalent and people finding remedies for them (Petrovska, 2012). Some of these diseases are cured naturally with the passage of time, and the rest need proper diagnosis and treatment. Indigenous systems of medicine have been followed by the ancient civilizations, and some of them are still very much in practice (Ravishankar & Shukla, 2007). With the passage of time and research inputs, man has been able to find the cause and cure for so many deadly diseases, but with today's fast-moving lifestyle, more complicated stress-related diseases are adversely affecting human life, and there is a dire need for proper health-care facilities for one and all in the society.

According to the WHO, good health is a resource of daily life and not only the purpose of living. It promotes a positive concept, which emphasizes our social and personal resources and develops our body's capacities. This was defined in 1986 and is still applicable. People with good health are happy and productive and are instrumental in building an economically strong nation. Economic growth in terms of numbers as is generally depicted, is a must but, when this growth leads to a better living standard for all the segments of the society, it is known as economic development. And this process of maintaining growth at a consistent level over the years is perceived as sustainable growth, according to the *Oxford Dictionary*, and sustainable growth leads to sustainable development. This is only possible when the general population is in good mental and physical health and is able to employ the available resources to some productive use that will lead to growth. A weak body or mind will not be able to concentrate in studies or work or even to think positively. Thus, we can say that a sustainable world requires sustainable growth, and a healthy population is always a prerequisite for sustainable growth. Sick people are a burden in the hospitals, devouring a lot of financial resources, while healthy people are seen in the factories, laboratories, playgrounds and conferences.

Computer aided diagnosis is a computer-based system that assists medical practitioners to take decisions in a very short span of time. Medical imaging deals with information in the form of image that the doctors and medical specialists use to examine and analyze for any form of abnormality in much less time. CAD has been a potential field of research for the last twenty years. However, it is a very complex field as it involves medication as well as engineering-related subjects. In order to widen the research overview of CAD, a literature survey with bibliometric analysis was conducted, and the study showed that CAD analysis has been filtered and defined as per the disease type and imaging technologies. This categorization was initiated with CAD for mammograms and further advanced to diseases related to the brain. Opportunities for the co-evolution of CAD research and imaging instruments – for example, the CAD of bones and pancreatic cancer were studied. The survey also said that there is a possibility of synergy with CAD and clinical decision support systems (Takahashi & Kajikawa 2017). With CAD, treatments become more meaningful, saving human lives and also enhancing the quality of lives.

3.2 Computer Aided Diagnosis

Computer aided detection systems assist medical practitioners in interpreting images relating to imaging techniques in x-rays, magnetic resonance imaging

(MRI), and ultrasound diagnostics. These systems create a lot of information that the radiologist or other concerned doctors use to examine and assess in a comprehensive manner, thereby supporting decisions taken by the medical professionals. Technologically advanced CAD systems are efficient for analyzing clinical data and gathering expertise that can further enhance the existing rules regarding diagnosis and enable such systems to improvise upon their performance over time. To ensure this, a proper feedback method should be there for these systems so that new knowledge can be drawn from different groups of data, based on their success and failures. The CAD systems can hence be considered as intellectual systems based on their learning capability (Obermeyer & Emanal, 2016). Intelligent CAD systems proficiently make use of artificial intelligence (AI), data mining and machine learning approaches to examine complex clinical data that can often be enormous in size. Such systems can be of great assistance in making correct decisions regarding clinical diagnosis in a wide range of diseases and medical conditions (Yanase, 2016; Giger, 2018).

The increasing research work with the help of diagnostic tools such as X-rays, ultrasounds or magnetic resonance imaging (MRI), has significantly increased our ability to understand the human anatomy and physiology over the years. This is evident when we compare the world's first edition of the oldest and most popular medical textbook, *The Merck Manual of Diagnosis and Therapy* (Beers, 1999) with its nineteenth edition. While the former was published in 1899 with 192 pages, the 2011 edition had 3,750 pages (Yanase, 2019; Porter et al., 2011). While many diseases have been successfully discovered with their treatment, the diagnosis of many others have become more difficult and complicated.

The two major facets of research in CAD are "detection" and "diagnosis" (Mansoor et al., 2015). Detection is the technique of locating the lesion region of the image thereby lessening the observational burden of the medical staff. While diagnosis is the technique used to identify the potential diseases. The aim is to provide medical practitioners with extra support. In most of the CAD systems, detection and diagnosis are strongly related. In the initial phase, the lesion is segmented from the normal tissue while, in the second phase, the lesion is properly assessed to produce a diagnosis (Huang et al., 2018).

3.3 Historical Background of Computer Aided Diagnosis

With the introduction of computers during the late 1950s, researchers working in areas related to the medical sciences took advantage of the opportunities of using computer aided diagnostic systems. In the initial stages, they worked with flow charts, pattern matching based on statistics, probability theory and knowledge bases in the CAD based decision-making process (Yanase &

Triantaphyllou, 2019). In the early 1970s, the first CAD systems, known as the "expert systems" in the medical field, were developed and mostly utilized for learning and teaching purposes. The MYCIN expert system (Shortliffe & Buchanan, 1975), the internist expert system (Miller, 1982) and the CADUCEUS expert system (Feigenbaum & McCorduck, 1984) are a few such examples. The experts in the field were focusing on developing fully automated CAD/expert systems during the initial days of early developments. These scientists were unrealistically optimistic in their expectations of computers. However, the available opportunities as well as shortcomings with the development of algorithms being used to resolve groups of important computational problems (Yanase, 2019), through a paper by Richard M. Karp titled, "Reducibility among Combinatorial Problems" (Karp, 1972), was soon clear to them. This realization of the existing limitations led researchers to work on innovative CAD systems based on advanced technology. Systematic research and development began on a large scale during the early 1980s at the Kurt Rossmann Laboratories for Radiologic Image Research in the Department of Radiology at the University of Chicago (de Azevedo-Marques et al., 2018). Since then, research on effects of digital images on radiologic diagnosis was going on full swing. Many researchers in Europe and the United States were involved in research and development of picture archiving and communication system (PACS). It was seen that, though PACS would be beneficial in administering radiologic images in the radiology department, and would also be cost-effective for hospitals, it seemed unlikely that PACS would be of some major clinical advantage to radiologists. Thus, a major question arose as to how the diagnosis of the radiologists would be assisted by the benefits of digital images and this led to the concept of computer aided diagnosis (Doi, 2007).

It was difficult to predict the success of the development of CAD schemes. Hence, it was decided to go for research in areas having potential to make significant impact on medicine if CAD could be developed in a successful manner. In those days, cardiovascular diseases, breast cancer and lung cancer were the prevailing areas of study in medicine. Hence, three main research projects were selected for detection and/or quantitative analysis of lesions involved in vascular imaging (Fujita et al., 1987), detection of lung nodules in chest radiographs (Giger et al., 1990) and detection of clustered micro calcifications in mammograms (Chan et al., 1987).

There are three main ideas from beginning until today on which the whole of the efforts on research and development of CAD are based. First and the foremost being that the developmental strategy of processes and techniques for detection and quantization of lesions in medical images is formed on the basis of the radiologist's perception involved in image readings, as they are the ones actually involved in radiologic diagnosis (Doi, 2006). An assumption was that there was a need for development of computer algorithms based on the perception of image readings. The second idea was based on the way the success of the efforts would be measured if CAD were successfully developed, and this would be evident with CAD being put to use on daily basis for routine clinical work all over the world. Hence, a decision was taken to produce and protect intellectual properties involved with the basic technologies related to CAD schemes and to promote them by communicating with medical industry personnel for commercial purposes. Thus, the first patent on CAD was filed in 1987 (Doi et al., 1987) and it became the most frequently cited patent in the area of CAD technology. The third idea was the promotion of wide acceptance of the concept called CAD and to make possible the distribution of CAD research at various institutions at the global level. It was realized that, in order to be successful, it was important to involve a large number of researchers from different institutions in different aspects of research in CAD. The spirit of competition prevailing among the CAD researchers should be changed to that of being colleagues promoting the same subject. Hence, for more than two decades from the initial days of CAD research, annual meetings of the Radiological Society of North America (RSNA) were held in Chicago, where they had large scientific exhibits. A detailed display of CAD research in chest, breast, and vascular imaging were presented at these exhibits. Invitations were sent in advance to 118 radiologists to bring their cases to the RSNA meeting in order to test the CAD scheme. This had promising results (Schiavon & Grigenti, 2008). Beginning in 1996, observer performance studies were carried out for five years, and a large number of researchers participated during the RSNA meetings for detection of various lesions of images in the chest with and without the computer output in order to let the radiologists have a firsthand experience of using CAD. This demonstrated and the usefulness of CAD (Abe et al., 2003), and helped in promoting the concept of CAD widely and quickly.

3.4 Applications of Computer Aided Diagnosis

All over the world, osteoporosis is one of the most serious health problems faced by the elderly people. The 2004 annual report of the International Osteoporosis Foundation clearly says that one out of every three women and one out of every five men who are 50 years or more in age, are suffering from osteoporosis. It is essential for early detection of fractures in the vertebral column, as thoracic and lumbar vertebrae are the most common areas of fractures related to osteoporosis. The risk of subsequent fractures increases five times once a vertebral fracture occurs (Black et al., 1999). Once a fracture is detected in the vertebral column, pharmacologic therapy with alendronate, salmon calcitonin nasal spray, or raloxifene are helpful in reducing the frequency of subsequent fractures (Black et al., 1996), with the use of CAD with lateral chest radiographs, the image interpretation of the radiologists can be improved to a great extent in the detection of vertebral fractures and lung nodules (Kasai et al., 2008).

The best tool available for screening for early detection of breast cancer is mammography. Breast cancer mortality rates have been reduced by 30–70 percent on effectively using mammographic screening (Desautels, May 2007). The radiologists are offered considerable assistance by computer-aided diagnosis for interpreting medical images. A CAD system studies the structure and characteristics of different tissues and applies this knowledge to diagnose abnormalities. Research was conducted on CAD system for diagnosing cancer in the breast by way of deep belief network (DBN) that detects breast mass region automatically and recognizes them as being malignant, benign or normal. The result of this research work proved that the performance of DBN is much better than the conventional classifiers. The accuracy level of a DBN for the multiple mass region of interest is 92.86 percent and that for the whole mass region of interest is, 90.84 percent which clearly reflects the viability of a DBN-based CAD system for application in breast cancer diagnosis (Al-antari et al., 2017).

Diabetic retinopathy can be managed using imaging techniques and has been proving its clinical importance. Retinal diseases can be documented over time, using Fundus photography and may gradually be more supportive in screening of retinopathy for diabetic patients (Baumal, 2018). Patients with media opacity, such as vitreous hemorrhage or cataract, can be helped to a great extent using B-scan ultrasonography (Skandesh et al., 2018). Fluorecein angiography (Gass et al., 1967) is of great help in visualizing retinal ischemia as well as leakage from retinal eovascularization and also in macular edema. Optical coherence tomography, an imaging technique proficient enough to evaluate retinal morphology with microscopic resolution (Huang et al., 1991), is a significant tool used to diagnose and manage diabetic macular edema. With the evolution of these technologies on a continued basis, their significance in managing and accurately diagnosing diabetic retinopathy has become increasingly evident (Salz & Witkin, 2015).

The chest radiographs and sputum cytology examinations traditionally used for screening for lung cancer were not very successful in reducing the mortality rate of this cancer. Biomolecular markers, autofluorescence bronchoscopy, low-dose spiral and high-resolution computed tomography, endobronchial ultrasonography, optical coherence tomography, confocal micro-endoscopy, positron emission tomography when used in combination with video-assisted thoracic surgery and intraluminal bronchoscopy treatments may be successful in providing new modalities to detect and cure lung cancer at the earliest stage possible (Sutedja, 2003).

There is a growing opportunity for computer-aided diagnostic (CAD) tools created by digital radiography. The Logicon Caries Detector (LCD) with the latest CAD software can play a significant role in improving the ability of the dentist in detecting and classifying caries. Dentists may be successful in finding two times as much early dentinal caries in need of restoration (or at least forceful noninvasive treatment) than in earlier days, while not unnecessarily treating other teeth that are in good health. With the help of LCD, dentists are able to acquire more information from dental digital radiography than with the naked eye, leading to better care of the patient (Tracy et al., 2011).

Due to its efficiency and safety, the ultra sound image has been widely used over the years for detecting different diseases (Drukker et al., 2002) such as breast cancer, liver cancer, gastroenteric diseases, cardiovascular diseases, spine curvature and muscle diseases. However, to be able to read ultrasound images, it requires extensive training and years of experience.

In this environment, CAD has become a significant tool for assisting radiologists in their diagnoses. In the 1960s, the original CAD system was used to diagnose tumor in the breast (Takahashi & Kajikawa, 2017). Medical practitioners and radiologists use the CAD system to conduct diagnosis from two views. The first is their past experience and the second is the opinion of the computer. Upon the proper application of the CAD system, there is considerable improvement in the accuracy of diagnosis, less time consumption and a remarkable decrease in the work load of doctors (Cheng et al., 2009).

The procedure to restore proper flow of blood through an artery is called angioplasty. This is done in a hospital by a specialized doctor with the help of computer aided diagnosis. A thin tube is threaded through a blood vessel in the arm or the groin up to the exact affected site in the artery. There is a tiny balloon in the end of the tube that helps in opening clogged arteries in the heart.

One such imaging test that allows doctors to check for diseases in one's body is the positron emission tomography (PET) scan. These are used in diagnosis and managing disorders in the central nervous system, including diseases such as depression, epilepsy, head trauma, Parkinson's disease and Azheimer's disease. There are tracers attached to compounds such as glucose, and by detection of radioactive glucose, the PET scan detects the areas in the brain utilizing glucose at the highest rates (Slough et al., 2016).

COVID-19 is a fast spreading deadly illness among people across the world which can be diagnosed by the help of chest X-Ray image analysis from MERS, SARS, and ARDS viral pneumonia. The best threshold value for the segmentation of a chest image is deduced by exploitation of Li's method and particle swarm intelligence. Then, Law's masks are applied to the segmented chest image for highlighting the secondary characteristics. Subsequently, nine different vectors of attributes are extracted from the Grey Level Co-occurrence Matrix (GLCM) representation of each Law's mask result. Finally, the decisions of ensemble classifiers are combined with the help of a weighted voting machine. An accuracy of 98.04% shown by the experimental findings, indicates that CAD scheme can be a promising COVID-19 diagnostic tool for medical practitioners (Mohammed et al., 2020).

3.5 Towards a Sustainable World

The most commonly used definition of the term sustainable development is from the Brundtland Report: "Sustainable development is development that meets the needs of the present days without compromising the ability of the future generations to meet their own needs." This means economic growth without abusing the free gifts of nature, which is actually meant for all living beings in the present as well as the generations to come. Depleting natural resources is the main cause of unbalance of minerals in air and water. Pollution in air and water caused by inefficient resource use (Emas, 2015) leads to numerous diseases among the people. An unhealthy population will physically, emotionally and also financially depend on the next generation for its needs. This vicious circle of unhealthy population is a curse for the society and will never lead to proper human development, which is the basis of sustainable development for the World.

Thus, in order to achieve sustainability at the global level, there is a need to have healthy and productive people all over the world. In 2015, 195 countries of the United Nations agreed to changing the world for the better by bringing together their respective governments, businesses, media houses, higher educational institutions, and non-governmental organizations working at their local level to make improvement in the lives of the people belonging to their country by the year 2030 (Global Movement, 2019). If implemented well, there will be considerable improvement in establishing good health and well-being for all people.

The three dimensions of sustainable development are environmental sustainability, social sustainability and economic sustainability (Mensah, 2019).

3.5.1 Environmental Sustainability

The term environmental sustainability can be inferred as maintaining the natural capital. It is a concept connected to both social as well as economic sustainability, yet quite separate from them (Morelli, 2011). Its main concern is whether environmental resources will be protected and maintained for future generations. It refers to the basic needs of human beings such as, good quality air, pollution-free water and hygienic food. Contaminated air and water or even unhygienic food cause various deadly diseases.

There are around 7 million premature deaths per year caused by air pollution as reported by the World Health Organization (WHO) in 2014. This amounts to one in eight of total deaths in the world, which proves that air pollution is the greatest environmental health risk in the world. It causes deadly diseases such as cancer, stroke and ischemic heart disease. Respiratory diseases, including acute respiratory infections and chronic obstructive pulmonary diseases, also develop due to inhalation of polluted air. Millions of lives can be saved by reducing air pollution. Noncommunicable diseases can be prevented by cleaning up the air we breathe. It also reduces risk of diseases among women and vulnerable groups, including children and the elderly, according to Flavia Bustreo, World Health Organization assistant director-general for Family, Women and Children's Health.

According to the US centre for Disease Control and Prevention (CDC), the root cause of waterborne diseases are pathogenic microbes that can be directly spread through contaminated water. Thus, we see that the environment has a direct impact on the health of the people.

If environmental sustainability is accepted as a major concern for one and all, the number of people affected by chronic diseases will be controlled to a great extent. It is like a complete circle whereby, if we want healthy people, we need to reduce environment pollution and maintain a sustainable world so that the natural resources are all balanced and future generations are also in good health. And healthy people are happy and think positive for the society in a way that further works for the betterment of the environment.

In recent times, fog computing has emerged as a practical solution for health care services as it facilitates continuously monitoring the health of patients in far-flung areas and detecting mosquito borne diseases at an early stage. It also reduces the latency and communication cost, which is a big concern of cloud computing. Wearable and IOT sensors are used to collect the relevant information for this purpose, and with the help of fog computing medical information is analyzed, categorized and shared among the user and health-care service providers. A similar coefficient is used to differentiate between various mosquito-borne diseases, depending upon the symptoms of the patient, and the fuzzy k-nearest neighbor approach is used to classify the user into the infected or uninfected category. Further, social network analysis is employed on the cloud layer to detect the outbreak of mosquito-borne diseases. The chances of the registered user to acquire or spread the disease is measured by computing the probability of disease outbreak, which is used to provide location-based awareness to prevent the epidemic (Varadarajan et al., 2019)

The occurrences of water borne diseases are not immediate disasters like erupting volcanoes. They grow in such a slow process that early detection would allow useful preventive measures. There are several problems such as the presence of large number of organisms with outbreak potential and geographical areas that prevent early detection of outbreaks. A typical laboratory recognizes several thousand organisms. Computers and sophisticated algorithms flag abnormal occurrences and supplement human judgment going beyond the traditional dependence on laboratory isolates. (Hunter et al., 2003)

Computer aided diagnosis of bacteria or viruses present in the air or water, or any object, can save life to a large extent. The novel Corona Virus 2019 has caused huge losses human life and economic recession across the globe. It was discovered during the end of 2019 as a harmful lung disease to in the city of Wuhan in China and since then has been rapidly spreading all over the world. The deep learning CAD system is reliable enough to achieve diagnostic performance on COVID-19 among all other lung diseases. It can be of great respite by detecting the infection and helping in its cure (Al-antari et al., 2017).

3.5.2 Social Sustainability

Social sustainability involves fostering the development of people, their communities and their cultures to help attain a meaningful life, with good healthcare facilities, proper education, gender equality, peace and stability across the globe (Saith, 2006). All these virtues in the society are possible only for people with good health. Health should be given the highest priority by oneself as well as by the respective government. People with good health can have a developing and happy society. Health includes both physical as well as mental health. Physical deterioration of a bodily system, if diagnosed at an early stage, can be checked with medicines or surgery, and the person's life span increased. Also, when a person is not in good mental health, his life gets disturbed, which affects his work as well his social relations. Also, his family becomes disturbed, and this negatively affects the society at large. This, if detected on time can be cured, and the person is able to live a healthy life.

Both physical and mental health can be taken care of by getting oneself thoroughly checked on an annual basis, and once a person crosses forty-five years of age, biannual checkups would help in timely diagnosis of deadly diseases in the body.

Positron emission tomography can be used to help diagnose and manage many central nervous system disorders. If diseases like depression can be detected and checked, the society can be saved from numerous suicides and from family breakups and job loss.

Cancer is one such life-threatening disease that disturbs the financial as well as emotional balance of the whole family of a patient irrespective of his social status and also leaves him in distress and depression. Cancer cells have a high metabolic rate when compared to non-cancerous cells and have high level of chemical activity. Because of this, Positron emission tomography (PET) scans are helpful both for detecting cancer, and for checking its spread, seeing if the treatment is effective and also for checking for a cancer recurrence.

Screening can detect early signs of cancer in people who do not experience any symptoms. This is important as treatment is likely to be more successful. Early detection can save life and property and lead to a less stressful society. There are national screening programs conducted in the UK for breast, cervical and bowel cancer irrespective of social status. These services save nine thousand lives each year (Cancer Screening, 2020). This can be adopted by other developing countries as well, because it can save lives and make society a better place.

Mammography makes use of low-dose x-rays to detect breast cancer at an early stage, much before any symptoms are felt by the women, even before the physician can detect them – when it is most treatable. The American Medical Association (AMA) and the American College of Radiology (ACR) advise mammograms on an annual basis for women above the age of forty. The National Cancer Institute (NCI) further adds that women with a personal or family history of breast cancer should discuss with their doctor about the right time to begin screening and, in that way, saving a fortune for the family.

The combined use of accurate and aggressive diagnostic and treatment techniques that validate screening and successfully bring down the mortality rate brings new hope for societies aspiring for development. Due to their past history of smoking, many people facing cardiovascular and pulmonary health problems and considered being at risk for surgical intervention can also benefit from CAD. The cost-effectiveness of lung cancer screening will strongly depend on the proper selection of the target population and the optimal application of these new techniques.

In spite of the prevailing epidemiological controversy with regards to the screening of lung cancer, it is viable to specifically define who are actually at risk and that, with the use of less invasive techniques, quality of life can be maintained and also the chances of survival of many lung cancer patients can be increased.

The term *sustainability* is inclusive of the term *happiness*. In July 2011, The United Nations General Assembly adopted the term *happiness* in order to redefine the term *development* with a holistic approach through Resolution 65/309. Out of 156 countries, Finland has been ranked the happiest country three times in a row. The parameters set for judging the same are per capita income, healthy and long lives for its people and social support. We can see that, in order be happy, one needs to be physically and mentally fit and only then can a person be an asset, contributing positively towards a sustainable world.

The government has a crucial role to play when good health of the people, both physical as well as mental, forms the basis of, and becomes a major contributor to, the economic growth of a nation. The longevity as well as the quality of human life matters. It becomes mandatory for policymakers to allocate funds for screening of the people above forty years of age and providing clean drinking water so that waterborne diseases are avoided. Also screening facilities free of cost to be made available in government run hospitals so that more people can avail them.

3.5.3 Economic Sustainability

Economic sustainability implies making optimal use of, and safeguarding and sustaining, both material and human resources in order to create long-term sustainable value. Maintenance of good health of the people in society is a major area of concern for economic sustainability. People who are physically fit are definitely more productive and contribute financially to their families and society at large. It is seen that medical expenses are huge and consume a major portion of a person's savings in times of illness and also drive people into heavy loans from relatives and friends in times of chronic diseases. This cost can be easily reduced and the money wisely utilized for productive purposes by proper monitoring of people's health at regular intervals. Scanning machines may initially pinch us in our pockets, but timely diagnosis of ailments and their proper treatment will definitely save us a fortune.

Some simple digital instruments like the oxymeter or glucometer or sphygmomanometer, if purchased for personal use and fortnightly readings duly recorded, can definitely help in monitoring one's blood pressure, sugar level, oxygen level in the blood and any alarming variation can be reported to the concerned doctor even before any symptoms appear, for further investigation and treatment. This will save both time and money and sometimes surgery can be avoided and treatments made easy.

Computer aided diagnosis facilitates and guides doctors for angiography, angioplasty and cardio echogram. Ultrasound, sonography or scanning and the electrocardiogram can be used to minimize time and cost.

A doctor–population ratio of 1:1000 is prescribed by the World Health Organization for proper medical requirements of the people. India achieved the ratio of 1.34 doctors for 1,000 Indian citizens as of 2017 (Kumar & Pal, 2018). Comparable figures in other countries are as follows: Australia, 3.374:1,000; Brazil, 1.852:1,000; China, 1.49:1,000; France, 3.227:1,000; Germany, 4.125:1,000; Russia, 3.306:1,000; United States, 2.554:1,000; Afghanistan, 0.304:1,000; Bangladesh, 0.389:1,000; and Pakistan, 0.806:1,000 (*Economic Times*, 2017). It is evident that developed nations have more than the required number of doctors and that they are in a better position to meet the needs of their people, who are not maintaining good health.

The medical equipment used for computer aided diagnosis are costly, and a diagnosis is an expensive affair for the common person. In order to make this facility available for the general public, a nation has to be financially very strong. Also, in order to benefit from CAD, people can acquire a medical insurance policy, because medical bills are very high even if a deadly disease is diagnosed in the early stages.

3.6 Implications of Computer Aided Diagnosis

From the above discussions it is evident that computer aided diagnosis cannot take the place of the doctor or any other specialist in the medical profession. It has a supportive but important role to play. It is the professional (generally a radiologist) who is actually responsible for finally interpreting a medical image. However, some CAD systems aim at detecting early signs of abnormality in patients which is certainly notpossible for experienced professionals. Thus, we can infer that early detection is a must for proper action and medications by the specialists concerned and can save a lot of money of the patient and avoid further complications. Also, with their personal touch and kind words, the professional practitioner lessens the anxiety of the patient and alleviates sufferings to a great extent.

Some CAD systems are deemed to be expert systems in medicine as they try emulating the decision-making process of diagnosis by the concerned medical specialists. Moreover, complex clinical data being massive in size, may be easily processed by CAD system in medicine so that they are able to gather new knowledge in order to improve their skills of diagnosis over time. Hence, they can be considered as intelligent systems as they steadily improve their performance using the feedback method (Yanase, 2019).

Computer aided diagnosis can be taken up as a business opportunity for those with enough capital. They install the expensive machinery and then provide employment opportunities to medical practitioners. They can have a strategic business partnership with some hospitals where they are a service provider by delivering timely and accurate results for the patients.

Reputed business organizations with a large number of employees enrolled, can include medical checkups as part of their human resources policies. On the basis of these records, they can do their manpower planning. Those employees who are under stress can be specially counseled and treated with necessary medications. Those diagnosed with other ailments can also be taken care of with proper financial assistance. In this way, employees get a sense of belonging and feel more loyal and respectful towards the organization. They become better employees trying to contribute their best towards the growth of the company. Those who are in good mental and physical health can be prepared for a bigger role in the organization with more responsibilities.

3.7 Limitations

With health industries and social institutions trying to contribute their bit towards a sustainable world, computer aided diagnosis is bounded by certain limitations.

Computer aided diagnosis cannot be used without the prescription of doctors who, with their knowledge and experience, know which test is to be conducted and which instrument to be used. One cannot go on trying with all the possible instruments as the human body should not be unnecessarily exposed to risks and, also, it would be a costly affair for the patient. Thus, we can say that no matter how accurate the diagnosis, it cannot match the knowledge and the experience of a qualified doctor.

Also, it requires experienced professionals (generally radiologists) who apply their knowledge for finally interpreting a medical image.

Computer aided diagnosis is an expensive affair and people with less income generally avoid getting scanned at regular intervals in order to check for some tumors or fissures. They can delay until some symptoms are surfaced, but by that time it might be too late for complete treatment.

The availability of some of these expensive instruments is, again, very limited. Sometimes for a particular test one has to travel to a different city and the travel expenses adding to the diagnosis cost can be unaffordable. At times people cannot get access to the limited number of computer-aided diagnostic equipment and ultimately have to suffer due to lack of timely diagnosis.

The maintenance of some of these instruments is a costly and difficult affair. Also, very soon an instrument might become outdated and procuring the latest one requires new investment.

Doctors become so dependent on these machines that, without the help of images or some report, they do not take any decision regarding the medication of the patient. In fact, doctors find confidence when their decisions are based on computer aided diagnosis.

The cost of a mammography in India ranges between Rs 1100 to Rs 3000. This is pretty high for people with less income, and women who are not financially independent generally avoid this extra annual expense. So, we see, the attitude of self-care needs to be ingrained in the minds of the general public.

3.8 Conclusion

With the existing pressure of population on these doctors and increase in the diseases, it is difficult to devote much time and attention to individual patients. Computer aided technology facilitates quick and accurate diagnosis. It saves both time and money and also helps avoid further complications and loss of life.

Thus, we see that with the help of CAD we can achieve the three Ps of sustainability: strong and healthy People, which makes for a Profitable and happy society on a Planet that has a clean and balanced environment.

3.9 The Road Ahead

Computer aided diagnosis is an interdisciplinary technology with a careful blend of artificial intelligence and computer vision with radiological and pathological image processing. These are systems that facilitate doctors with proper interpretation of images related to the medical field. This imparts great relief to the stressed minds of the patients and their loved ones by providing accurate details regarding the size of the tumor, exact location or the existence of cancer cells in the body much ahead of any symptom experienced by the person. This way we can see that research has really done wonders, and people are able to fight the deadly diseases and live an enriching life for their family members and other dependents. CAD system also exhibits its ability and reliability in diagnosing COVID-19 along with other lung diseases.

Timely detection of fatal tumors can save so much of agony and hard-earned money of the patient. With more and more research in this field, we can overcome the cruel streak of sickness prevalent in society, maladies that hamper growth and also costs a major share of scarce resources.

References

Abe, Hiroyuki, Heber MacMahon, Roger Engelmann, Qiang Li, Junji Shiraishi, Shigehiko Katsuragawa, Masahito Aoyama, Takayuki Ishida, Kazuto Ashizawa, Charles E. Metz & Kunio Doi. (2003). Computer-aided Diagnosis in Chest Radiography: Results of Large- Scale Observer Tests at the 1996–2001. *Radiographics*, 23(1): 255–265.

Al-antari, Mugahed A., Cam-Hao Hua, Jaehun Bang & Sungyoung Lee. (n.d.). Fast Deep Learning Computer-Aided Diagnosis against the Novel COVID-19 Pandemic from Digital Chest X-ray Images. *Research Square.*

Al-antari, Mugahed A., Mohammed A. Al-masni, Sung-Un Park, JunHyeok Park, Mohamed K. Metwally, Yasser M. Kadah, Seung-Moo Han & Tae-Seong Kim. (2017). An Automatic Computer-Aided Diagnosis System for Breast Cancer in Digital Mammograms via Deep Belief Network. *Journal of Medical and Biological Engineering*, 443–456.

Baumal, Caroline R.(2018). Imaging in Diabetic Retinopathy. In Caroline R. Baumal and Jay S. Duker, *Current Management of Diabetic Retinopathy* (pp. 25–36). Elsevier. St. Louis, MI.

Beers, Mark H. (1999). *The Merck Manual of Diagnosis and Therapy*. Merck Research Laboratories, Division of Merck & Co. Whitehouse Station, NJ.

Black, Dennis. M., Nigel K. Arden, Lisa Palermo, Jim Pearson, Steven R. Cummings. & Study of Osteoporotic Fractures Research Group. (1999). Prevalent Vertebral Deformities Predict Hip Fractures and New Vertebral Deformities but Not Wrist Fractures. *Journal of Bone and Mineral Research*, 14(4): 821–828.

Black, Dennis M., Steven R. Cummings, David B. Karpf, Jane A. Cauley, Desmond E. Thompson, Michael C. Nevitt, Douglas C. Bauer, Harry K. Genant, William L. Haskell, Robert Marcus, Susan M. Ott, James C. Torner, Sara A. Quandt, Theodore F. Reiss & Kristine E. Eensrud. (1996). Randomised Trial of Effect of Alendronate on Risk of Fracture in Women with Existing Vertebral Fractures. Fracture Intervention Trial Research Group. Lancet 348(9041): 1535–1541.

Chan, Heang-Ping, Kunio Doi, Simranjit Galhotra, Carl J. Vyborny, Heber Macmahon, Peter M. Jokich. (1987). Image Feature Analysis and Computer-Aided Diagnosis in Digital Radiography. I. Automated Detection of Micro Calcifications in Mammography. *Medical Physics*, 14(4): 538–548.

Cheng, Heng-Da, Juan Shan, Wen Ju & Yanhui Guo. (2009). Automated Breast Cancer Detection and Classification Using Ultrasound Images. *Pattern Recognition*, 43(1): 299–317.

de Azevedo-Marques, Paulo Mazzoncini, Arianna Mencattini, Marcello Salmeri & Rangaraj M. Rangayyan (eds). (2018). *Medical Image Analysis and Informatics: Computer-Aided Diagnosis and Therapy*. Taylor & Francis Group.

Desautels, l. May. (2006). A review of computer-aided diagnosis of breast cancer: Toward the detection of subtle signs. *Journal of the Franklin Institute*, 312–348.

Doi, Kunio, Heang-Ping Chan. & Maryellen L. Giger. (1987). Method and System for Enhancement and Detection of Abnormal Anatomic Regions in a Digital Image. PAT: US4907156.

Doi, Kunio. (2006). Diagnostic Imaging Over the Last 50 Years: Research and Development in Medical Imaging Science and Technology. *Physics in Medicine and Biology*, 51(13): R5–27.

Doi, Kunio. (2007). Computer-Aided Diagnosis in Medical Imaging: Historical Review, Current Status and Future Potential. *PubMed*, 198–211.

Drukker, Karen, Maryellen L. Giger, Karla Horsch, Matthew A. Kupinski, Carl J. Vyborny, Ellen B. Mendelson. (2002). Computerized Lesion Detection on Breast Ultrasound. *Medical Physics*, 29(7): 1438–1446.

Emas, Rachel. (2015). *The Concept of Sustainable Development: Definition and Defining*. Florida: GDSR.

Feigenbaum, Edward A. & Pamela McCorduck. (1984). *The Fifth Generation. Signet*; ISBN-13: 978-0451152640.

Fujita, Hiroshi, Kunio Doi, Laura E. Fencil & Kok Gee Chua. (1987). Image Feature Analysis and Computer-Aided Diagnosis in Digital Radiography. 2. Computerized Determination of Vessel Sizes in Digital Subtraction Angiography. *Medical Physics*, 14(4): 549–556.

Gass, J. Donald M., Raymond J. Sever, Dixie Sparks, Joseph Goren. (1967). A Combined Technique of Fluorescein Funduscopy and Angiography of the Eye. *Archives of Opthalmology*, 78(4): 455–461.

Giger, Maryellen Lissak, Nicholas Ahn, Kunio Doi, Heber MacMahon & Charles E. Metz. (1990). Computerized Detection of Pulmonary Nodules in Digital Chest Images: Use of Morphological Filters in Reducing False-Positive Detections. *Medical Physics*, 17(5): 861–865.

Giger, Maryellen Lissak. (2018). Machine Learning in Medical Imaging. *Journal of the American College of Radiology*, 15(3): 512–520.

Global Movement – Government Transparency: The Sustainable Development Goals (SDG). (2019). Retrieved June 28, 2020, from https://worldtop20.org/global-movement.

Huang, David, Eric A. Swanson, Charles P. Lin, Joel S. Schuman, William G. Stinson, Warren Chang, Michael R. Hee, Thomas Flotte, Kenton Gregory, Carmen A. Puliafito, et al. (1991). Optical Coherence Tomography. *Science*, 254(5035): 1178–1181.

Huang, Qinghua, Zhang Fan & Li Xuelong. (2018). Machine Learning in Ultrasound Computer-Aided Diagnostic Systems: A Survey. *Biomed Research International*, 2018 Mar 4; 2018: 5137904.

Hunter, Paul Raymond, Michael Waite & Elettra Ronchi (eds). (2003). *Drinking Water and Infectious Disease: Establishing the Links*. London: IWA Publishing.

Karp, Richard M. (1972). *Reducibility among Combinatorial Problems*. New York: Plenum Press.

Kasai, Satoshi, Feng Li, Junji Shiraishi & Kunio Doi. (2008). Usefulness of Computer-Aided Diagnosis Schemes for Vertebral Fractures and Lung Nodules on Chest Radiographs. *American Journal of Roentgenology*, 191: 260–265.

Kumar, Raman & Ranabir Pal. (2018). India Achieves WHO Recommended Doctor Population Ratio: A Call for Paradigm Shift in Public Health Discourse! *Journal of Family Medicine and Primary Care*, Sep–Oct; 7(5), 841–844.

Mansoor, Awais, Ulas Bagci, Brent Foster, Ziyue Xu, Georgios Z. Papadakis, Les R. Folio, Jayaram K. Udupa & Daniel J. Mollura. (2015). Segmentation and Image Analysis of Abnormal Lungs at CT: Current Approaches, Challenges, and Future Trends. *Radiographics*, 35(4): 1056–1076.

Miller, Randolph A., Harry E. Pople, Jack D. Myers. (1982). Internist-I, an Experimental Computer-Based Diagnostic Consultant for General Internal Medicine. *New England Journal of Medicine*, 307(8): 468–476.

Mohammed, Suhaila N., Fatin Sadiq A. & Yasmin A. Hassan. (2020). Automatic Computer Aided Diagnostic for COVID-19 Based on Chest X-Ray Image and Particle Swarm Intelligence. *International Journal of Intelligent Engineering and Systems*, 13(5): 63–73.

Morelli, John. (2011). Environmental Sustainability: A Definition for Environmental Professionals. *Journal of Environmental Sustainability*, 1(2011). DOI: 10.14448/jes.01.0002.

Obermeyer, Ziad & Ezekiel J. Emanual. (2016). Predicting the Future – Big Data, Machine Learning, and Clinical Medicine. *New England Journal of Medicine*, 375: 1216–1219.

Petrovska, B. Bauer. (2012). Historical Review of Medicinal Plants' Usage. *Pharmacognosy Review*, 6(11): 1–5.

Porter, Robert S., Justin L. Kaplan & Barbara P. Homeier (eds). (2011). *The Merck Manual Home Health Handbook*. Hoboken, NJ. John Wiley.

Ravishankar, Bharat & Vinay J. Shukla. (2007). Indian Systems of Medicine: A Brief Profile. *African Journal of Traditional, Complementary and Alternative Medicines: AJTCAM*, 4: 319–337.

Saith, Ashwani. (2006). From Universal Values to Millennium Development Goals: Lost in Translation. *Development and Change*, 37(6): 1167–1199.

Salz, David A. & Andre J. Witkin. (2015). Imaging in Diabetic Retinopathy. *Middle East African Journal of Ophthalmology*, 22: 145–150.

Schiavon, Francesco & Fabio Grigenti. (2008). *Radiological Reporting in Clinical Practice*. Milan: Springer.

Shortliffe, Edward H. & Bruce G. Buchanan. (1975). A Model of Inexact Reasoning in Medicine. *Mathematical Biosciences*, 2(3–4): 351–379.

Skandesh B. M., Mohan Kumar & Sreenivasa Raju N. (2018). Role of High Resolution Sonography (B-SCAN) in the Evaluation of Posterior Segment Lesions of Eye. *International Journal of Contemporary Medicine Surgery and Radiology*, 3(3): C11–C16.

Slough, Coutney, Shane C. Masters, Robin A. Hurley, & Katherine H. Taber. (2016). Clinical Positron Emission Tomography (PET) Neuroimaging: Advantages and Limitations as a Diagnostic Tool. *Journal of Neuropsychiatry and Clinical Neurosciences*, 28, 67–71.

Sutedja, Tom G. (2003). New Techniques for Early Detection of Lung Cancer. *European Respiratory Journal*, 57s–55s.

Takahashi, Ryohei & Yuya Kajikawa. (2017). Computer-aided Diagnosis: A Survey with Bibliometric Analysis. *International Journal of Medical Informatics*, 101: 58–67.

Tracy, Kyle D., Bradley A. Dykstra, David C. Gakenheimer, James P. Scheetz, Stephani Lacina, William C. Scarfe & Allan G. Farman. (2011). Utility and Effectiveness of Computer-Aided Diagnosis of Dental Caries. *General Dentistry*, 59: 136–144.

Varadarajan, Vijayakumar, Devarajan Malathi, Vairavasundaram Subramaniyaswamy, Palani Saravanan & Logesh Ravi. (2019). Fog Computing-based Intelligent Healthcare System for the Detection and Prevention of Mosquito-borne Diseases. *Computers in Human Behavior*, 100: 275–285.

Yanase, Juri & Evangelos Triantaphyllou. (2019). A Systematic Survey of Computer-Aided Diagnosis in Medicine: Past and Present Developments. *Expert Systems with Applications*.

4

Applications of Generative Adversarial Network on Computer Aided Diagnosis

Chandrani Singh and Sourav De

CONTENTS

4.1 Introduction

Digital imaging and image analysis approaches otherwise known as Computer Aided Diagnosis or Computer Aided Detection have created a competitive edge with respect to the speed and performance over human-based image analysis. Computer aided detection (CADe) and computer aided diagnosis (CADx) are evolving technologies that enable radiologists to infer from medical images. While CADe can help medics to identify a cancer, CADx enables radiologists to conclude whether there is a need for tissue culture from the region currently under investigation and subsequent analysis of the same [1]. CADe and CADx algorithms differ in the input data and the output. In actuality, while CADe identifies the location of malignancy, the computer aided diagnosis certifies whether a known laceration is malignant. Commercial computer-aided detection techniques have enabled radiologists to accurately detect and improvise the recall rate and in recent times has been approved by US Federal Governmental Department of Health and Human Service. However until now commercial computer-aided diagnosis has not envisaged sizeable integration into the clinical space, owing to the limitations in enhancing CAD performance coupled with the improvised methods of implementing CAD. Computer aided detection and computer aided diagnosis have been evolving consistently, and in recent times many researches are being carried out that have made phenomenal progress in terms of improvising on accuracy and performance. Computer aided diagnosis is a program that provides morphologic analysis, and such systems were developed to overcome the discrepancy and difference in the views of the observer with an objective to improve the competence of the radiologists in the analysis of the images and provide substantive evidence of malignancy in the tissues. The functional component of a Computer Aided Detection and Diagnosis system is as follows [2]: With reference to image sizing in Figure 4.1, the digital images are adjusted to the window width and level to gain extra information, and adaptive histogram equalization is a technique that adjusts the width and level of each sub area under consideration. The step of extraction under the component of CAD can otherwise be stated as digital subtraction, whereby a normal CT scan differs from a contrast CT and the resulting image shows non-zero values if and only if there

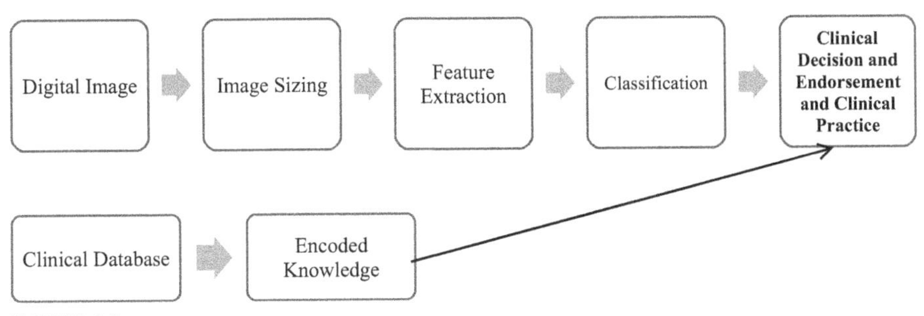

FIGURE 4.1
Functional Components of Computer Aided Detection/Diagnosis.

exists a difference, and this subtraction technique has been applied to chest radio graphs and mammograms, magnetic resonance imaging (MRI), positron emission tomography (PET), and single-photon emission computed tomography (SPECT). With reference to the classification/pattern recognition, both syntactic and statistical pattern recognition are used to set the rules for classification succeeded by classification of cases into categories, and both these techniques would be used to aid in differential diagnosis. Neural Network on other hand includes examinations from multiple time points and is classified as also a pattern-recognition technique. While the weights associated across the neurons and levels can become altered, the problem of noise and over fitting have to be handled carefully. The information modelling probabilities aim at collating data/information that is specific and generic to patients in order to improve on the accuracy and are specifically attributed to information on the images.

While Figure 4.1 describes a generic framework for computer aided detection or diagnosis, the below framework is specific to detection of prostrate carcinoma using MRI. The images on the left of Figure 4.2 are the MRI modalities such as T2 Weighted MRI, DCE MRI, DW MRI, ADC Map, MRSI and so forth. The T2 Weighted MRI gives the best detection of the prostrate zonal anatomy and is also used for localization and staging. Dynamic contrast enhanced (DCE) MRI exhibits a likeness of former and later gadolinium images by administering gadolinium-based contrast medium, but is usually incapable of identifying the prostate cancer. In comparison, Magnetic Resonance Spectroscopic Imaging (MRSI) displays the lower citrate levels and higher levels of choline of prostate cancer in comparison to non-malignant tissue.

All these images act as the input data, and under image regularization three steps are performed as follows: Preprocessing, Segmentation and Registration. The regularized images are then subjected to CAD(e) and CAD(x). The detection of Region of Interest is done in the first phase as in Figure 4.3, whereas in CAD(x), feature detection, extraction and classification

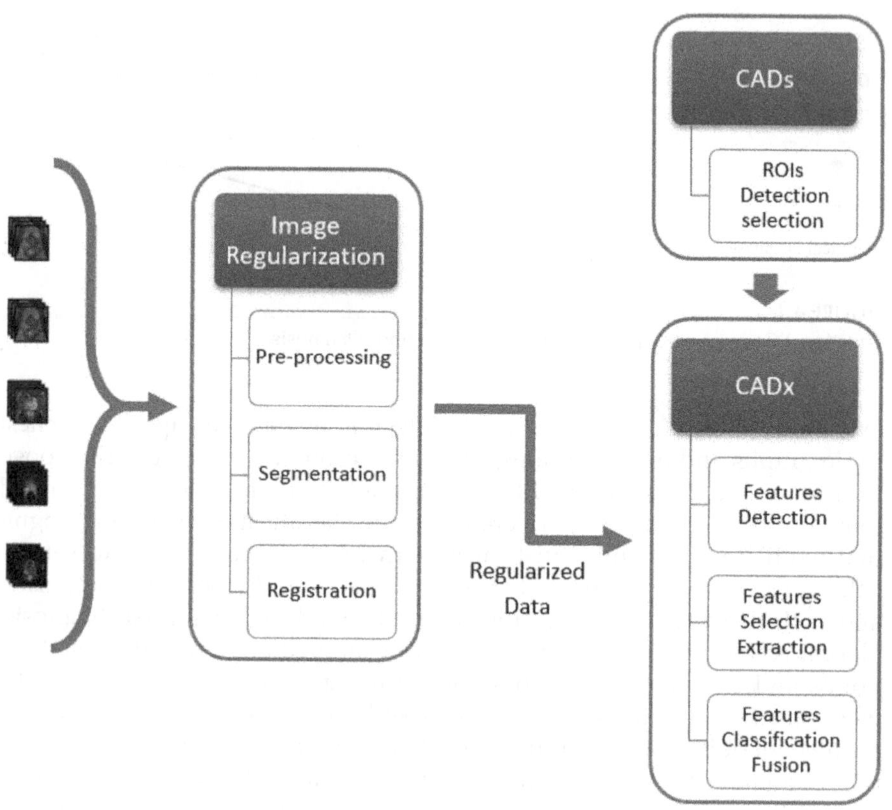

FIGURE 4.2
A CAD Framework Based on MRI to Identify Prostate Cancer.

is done. Currently the commercial CAD x that are available in the market as Image Checkers are as follows:

- *EmphaSize* – Here the marks are exhibited in various sizes, and they normally correlate to prominent features in a mass or lesion and also in calcification clusters. When certain regions of interest exude greater prominence of features, the CAD marks enlarge. Here the key features evaluated are signal intensity, calcification shape and number in that region of interest. For evaluation of masses, degree of spiculation, lesion shape, contrast to surrounding tissue, lesion interior, and edge texture are considered. For a region containing both lesion and calcification, the Image Checker produces a Malc mark and scales it depending on the prominence.
- *PeerView* – The reason why the Image Checker CAD algorithm marked a particular region and outlining of that doubtful region to enable the radiologists to envisage and investigate the specific structures is based

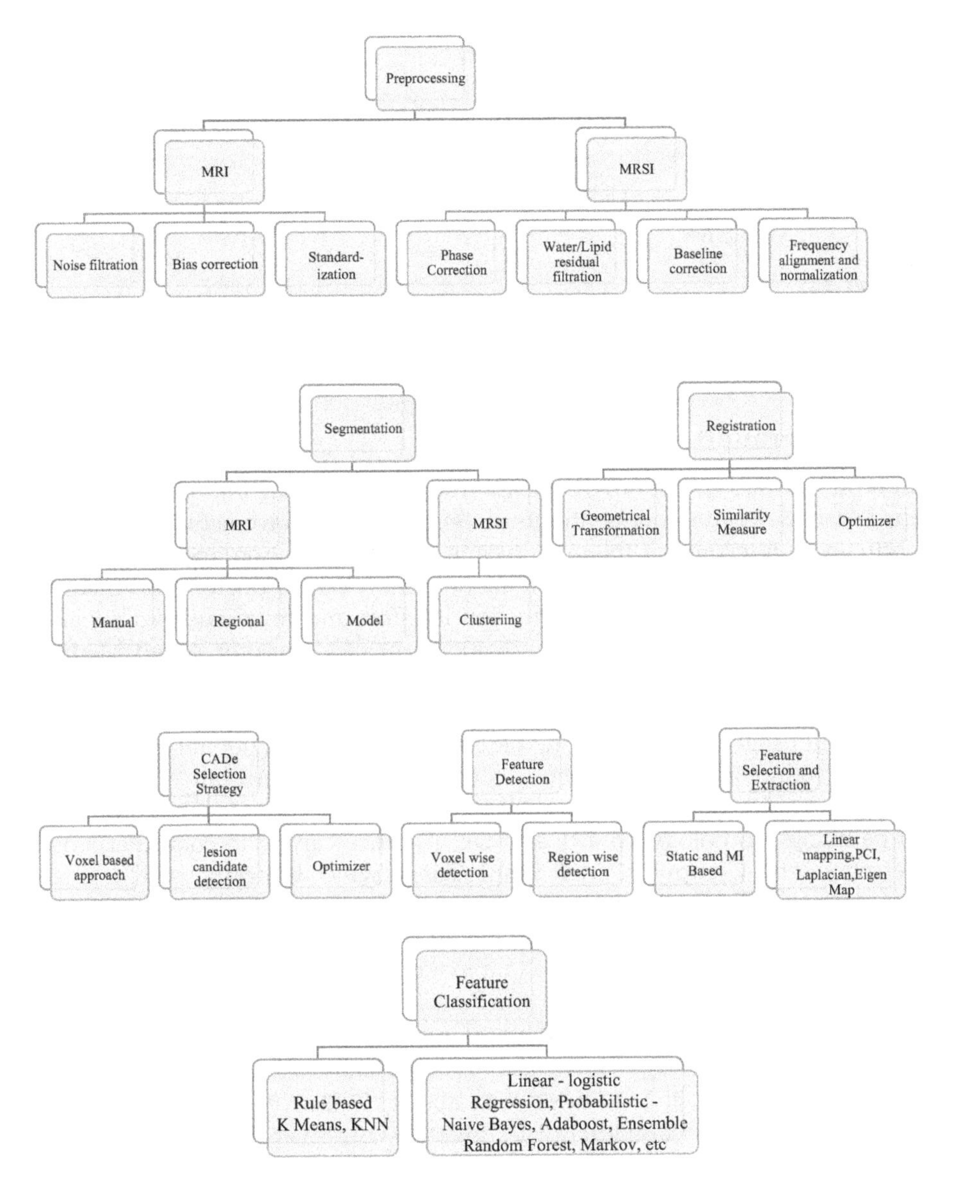

FIGURE 4.3
Phase Description of CAD Framework.

on their margin, shape and interior characteristics. Detected micro-calcifications are highlighted so the radiologist can determine the number, shape and distribution.

- *LesionMetrics* – on the other hand measures the position of distortion and goes into the detail of identifying from the portion, the fraction that is speculated.

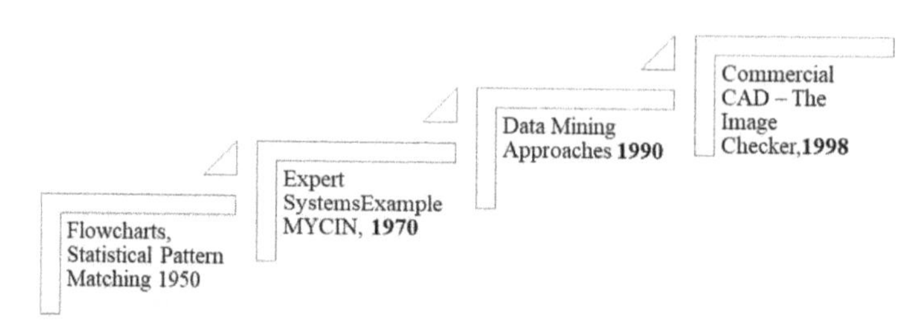

FIGURE 4.4
Evolution of Computer Aided Detection/Diagnosis.

4.2 Background

Computer aided detection/diagnosis systems have come into prominence in the last few decades, are continuously evolving and have achieved relevant accuracy in interpreting the medical images. The evolution and the progression in this segment have brought about great relief for doctors and medical practitioners with substantial reduction in effort and time rendered for analysis of the output. The phased advancement of Computer Aided Medical Diagnosis can be depicted by Figure 4.4. CAD systems are mainly used to process and diagnose digital images and highlight the abnormalities identified. Their usage is well established in identification of congenital heart defect, diabetic retinopathy, malignancy in colon, lung, breast, prostate and so forth. Computer aided diagnosis/detection is interdisciplinary and is the confluence of pathology, radiology, AI, ML and DL. Another variant to computer aided detection is the Computer Aided Simple Triage, which is mostly used for emergency diagnostic imaging whereby a quick diagnosis of a life-threatening condition is required. CAD systems to date cannot identify the suspicious features in totality, and the three measures that in a major way identify the robustness of CAD are Sensitivity, Specificity and Absolute Detection Rate.

The classification algorithms that are used especially for diagnosis consist of Naive Bayesian Classifier, Support Vector Machine, Principal Component Analysis and Artificial Neural Network, using which every Region of Interest (ROI) is analyzed. Digital images are subjected to extensive analysis by CAD systems through a series of steps such as Pre-processing, Segmentation, Analysis and Classification of ROI above a certain threshold.

4.3 Computer Aided Detection and Research Progression

Computer Aided Detection (CAD) is a technology that assists in reducing the false negative rates of interpreting the medical images by the radiologists. In other words, it can be defined as a pattern recognition software that detects abnormalities, the output of which is analyzed by the radiologists. Computer aided detection is FDA and CE approved for digital mammography with respect to screening and diagnosis. CAD algorithms search for distortions, calcifications and asymmetries when conducting digital mammography while, for chest CT scans, CAD systems try to evaluate pulmonary densities. A CAD mark as perceived by the radiologist, that which is TP (True Positive), does not require any investigation, whereas a false negative might require specific interpretations of the radiologist and should be subjected to thorough investigations.

4.4 Implementation and Assessment of Clinical CAD

The CAD algorithms require conversion of analog images to its digital counterpart or can analyze the images in the digital format directly. The clinical interpretations are arrived at by first analyzing the films using the manual mode, which is usually done by the radiologist, and then the digital image is served as an input to the CAD software, and areas that are marked by the software are re-reviewed by the radiologists. Current computer aided detection systems have the limitations of not being able to mark all the areas in the image, where action is required, and these systems are prone to generate more false positives than true positives. Hence, there is a dire need to assess whether the CAD marked area should be subjected to further evaluation or not. A Computer Aided Detection System's robustness can be evaluated either by using it in an environment with a substantial quantity of test data or by assessing radiologists' performance based on the support rendered by CAD. In addition, they can be evaluated by scoring on the sensitivity and specificity, where sensitivity is defined as the percentage of cases that are confirmed to be positive and have also been marked by the CAD system, whereas the number of false CAD marks identified is the specificity. To evaluate CAD systems along sensitivity and specificity, a large number of truth cases should be used to establish the statistical significance first, and that will also act as a basis to evaluate various CAD systems based on their performance [4]. CAD evaluations can also be done by comparing setups that have no CAD support vis-a-vis setups that have strong and consistent CAD support. Here an important limitation is that in many cases the radiologists may over- or under-call the reviewed cases. But the best results are achieved when the disease detection first happens manually and then with the CAD intervention and, subsequently, recall rates are monitored. However, percentage change in disease detection with CAD intervention should be less than the percentage change exuded in the detection through utilization of the recall rate.

In the succeeding section, the application of AI, ML and DL in CAD has been considered for discussion. Several machine-learning algorithms contributing to improvised accuracy with a focus on sensitivity, specificity, absolute detection out-performing traditional CAD, thus substantially justifying the research progression in the said domain. Table 4.1 represents the study of the intelligent applications built for computer aided detection.

Recent breakthroughs in artificial intelligence (AI) have direct implications for computer aided detection and diagnosis (CAD(e) and/or CAD(x)) specifically in the field of medical science. The aim is to showcase the artificial intelligence enabled detection systems, which are of great support to the radiologists. They help in identifying the location within the ROI, that is, the region of interest, of carcinomas found in the different parts of the body, be it the lungs, colon, prostrate, breasts and so forth, or any other symptomatic condition the patient encounters. An automated computer aided diagnosis (CAD) system can act as a real time decision support system for the medics and can verify and validate the radiologist's interpretation. In addition, complementary handcrafted features, like location, context features and temporal changes added to the CNN also help to improvise the performance up to the standards of a radiologist. Measures or parameters that have been frequently used to evaluate the operation of the algorithms that can perform the find or the selection are as follows: The two very popular measures used to assess the algorithms correctly are Sensitivity and Specificity, those which are described in the succeeding sections. **Sensitivity** is the probability of correctly identifying the positive cases among the diseased candidates, whereas the probability that tests would give negative results in the case of people who are healthy is termed **Specificity** and will be used throughout the literature. Another type of score commonly used to check the robustness of the computer aided diagnosis is the AUC-ROC curve where ROC (Receiver Operating Characteristics) is a probability curve, and Area Under the Curve (AUC) represents the measure of distinctiveness with respect to the classes that are created. A good model is represented by a higher AUC. The subsequent sections consist of results and discussions that best portray the usage of these measures to identify the lesion localization.

Several of the deep learning algorithms like CNN, RESNET taken into consideration during the researches conducted, showcase improved specificity with inclusion of location and context features, whereas algorithms like Conditional Regression have been found to present better interpretation of images when infused in the CAD systems. The specificity and sensitivity results for bi-recurrent neural networks have shown a performance even close to 100 percent, both in cases of arterial fibrillation detection and in cases of colonoscopy, justifying the beneficial intervention through adoption of AI and ML in computer aided diagnosis. But the limitations that prevent getting FDA approval construe various medical equipment producing the images, and these images being assessed by machine learning algorithms, for which results are portrayed differently.

TABLE 4.1

Literature Study of Usage of AI/ML Techniques in CAD(e)

Year	Authors	Objective	Design Methodology	Setting	Participants and Body Region	Measures and Outcome	Results
2015	Lehman *et al.* [5]	Performance measurement of Digital Screening Mammography with and without CAD(e)	Mammography Image Interpretation using models to evaluate the performance	With CAD – 4 Lakh plus images considered Without CAD – 1 Lakh plus images considered	Women, Female Breasts and 271 Radiologists	Mammography performance with respect to specificity, sensitivity, interval cancers absolute detection were modeled **Logistic regression** used to account for correlation between interpretations of the same radiologist and **Conditional logistic regression** to compare interpretations by radiologists with and without CAD	Sensitivity, Specificity and Absolute detection rate did not improve with CAD and did not improve intra radiologist performance
2015	Lemaitre *et al.* [5]	Provide a comprehensive review focusing on the different phases, the work-flow of a computer-aided DeDx System	Comprehensive Review using literature on CAD workflow		Literature Study based on MRI Modality, studied zones and CAD stages Prostrate (Men)	Evaluation measures were AUC-ROC, Sensitivity, Specificity, FROC extends ROC analysis to a region-based level, and Dice Coefficient – Accurately measure	Results reported with respect to sensitivity, Specificity, AUC-ROC and vary between 71 pc to 97 pc with different brands of MRI Scanner

(continued)

TABLE 4.1 (Continued)

Literature Study of Usage of AI/ML Techniques in CAD(e)

Year	Authors	Objective	Design Methodology	Setting	Participants and Body Region	Measures and Outcome	Results
2017	Pirouzbak *et al.* [6]	Prepossessing of the mammogram images using the contour let transform and a new neural network topology of layers adapted for the task of breast cancer detection	Stage 1- consists of pre-processing of data and Stage 2 consists of feeding the data to the network topology with 1,07,257 and 2 neurons	Computer with a Core i7-6500 + HQ, 2.6GHz × 8processor and 30 + GB of RAM and 300 mammograms	Women Female breasts	Convolutional Neural Network performed 4000 iterations and executed 100 pc accuracy	Preprocessing the mammogram image to remove artifact, and enhanced contrast by means of the NSCT, feeding the image to a deep neural network. Preprocessing facilitated the filters in the convolutional layers to classify correctly the images, even with a small training set.
2017	Kooi *et al.* [7]	Comparing Mammography CAD systems where manually designed features are considered vis-à-vis CNN's That can read mammograms independently			Women Female Breasts	Convolution Neural Network shows improved specificity with inclusion of location and context features and outperforms traditional CAD at high sensitivity	No difference between CNN and certified screening radiologist and outperforming traditional CAD.

2018	Qin *et al.* [8]	Usage of CAD in spotting the pulmonary nodules, identifying TB, and interstitial lung diseases. Laying a special emphasis on the algorithmic principles, the dataset used for study, the performance assessment parameters and the findings	Data-set collection, image preprocessing followed by single and multiple diseases	Trained on 45000 images of which around 11000 DI-COM cases are from Korea Tuberculosis Institute(KIT), 7020 cases from Montgomery County Dataset, Maryland US. and remaining from JSRT and Shenzen dataset	Mix of male and female with chest radiograph	Usage of RESNET,CHEXNET CNN have exhibited greater degree of accuracy from 65 pc to 92 pc	A survey article that justifies and exhibits the usage of AI to improve on the diagnostic accuracy.
2019	Fujita *et al.* [9]	To accurately detect fibrillations and flutter using 8-layer CNN	Basic data normalization for implementation of the proposed model and designing two relative models to validate the classification performance using 10-fold cross-validation	Python Programming and Google Tensor Flow deep learning libraries Database used -MITBIH AF database (AFDB) and the MIT-BIH arrhythmia database (MITDB)	Both gender, Heart	Modelling to achieve high specificity, sensitivity and accuracy. The number of layers for the Bi-Recurrent Neural Network was constrained to 2	The accuracy, specificity, and sensitivity of the model are as follows: 98.8%, 98.6%, and 98.9% on the AFDB database and the improvised performance is noted as 99.4%, 99.1%, with the MITDB database

(continued)

TABLE 4.1 (Continued)

Literature Study of Usage of AI/ML Techniques in CAD(e)

Year	Authors	Objective	Design Methodology	Setting	Participants and Body Region	Measures and Outcome	Results
2020	Misawa *et.al* [10]	To develop An artificial intelligence enabled polyp detection system and to confirm its operation using a sizeable colonoscopy video database that is made accessible to public	Development and training and validation of the AI impregnated Deep Learning system with annotation by endoscopist on the presence and absence and the location of the polyp	56,668 independent colonoscopy images	Both the gender participated, Colon	1405 videos were found for the substantiation. Of these,797 contained at least one polyp and 13 videos, negative for polyps were randomly extracted. Total number of frames considered were 152,560 of which 49,799 were positive and 102,761 were negative	Frame based analysis exuded 90.5% sensitivity, 93.7% specificity The per-polyp sensitivities for all, small, projected, and flat polyps were over 98.0%, respectively

4.5 Application of Machine Learning and Deep Learning in Computer Aided Detection

4.5.1 Generative Adversarial Network – the State of the Art Architecture

Generative Adversarial networks are built upon the machine learning frameworks that consist of two NN's (neural networks); one is the generator and the other, the discriminator. The former can generate new images from the trained data set, while the latter discriminates between the original and the generated ones. The discriminator neural net relies on the initial training set to achieve the desired accuracy, while the generator is allocated a random input, and the candidates generated are presented to the discriminator to distinguish between the original and the synthesized images. Generative Adversarial Network Models can be scaled up in terms of model capacity, or can exude incremental growth during training, thus ensuring learnability and generation of high-quality images. This acts as a strong indicator to explore further the capabilities of GAN particularly in the health-care segment. Here, both the neural networks use the concept of back propagation to build on their own level of accuracy, that is, the generator model, through successive refinements, builds images that are very similar to the trained set, while the discriminator model achieves the desired expertise in the flagging of the synthesized images. To describe this more in detail, a generator model produces false images by taking into consideration some non-validated information. With support from the Discriminator, the model begins creating images of a particular class that appears authentic, and the Discriminator tells the generator the resemblance to the genuine image and helps to identify the false images. The work-flow sequence of GAN as shown in Figure 4.5 is as follows:

Insight on Generative Adversarial Network and its application in the last five years presents the fact that the said framework has envisaged a high degree of utilization, greater accuracy and improvement in performance, justifying the current fitment and the emerging range of the said techniques in the field of computer aided diagnosis and pattern recognition.

4.5.2 Generative Adversarial Network – Evaluation Methodology

Generative adversarial networks are deep learning models that are not trained with an objective loss function, unlike others, and certain qualitative and quantitative techniques are used to assess the performance of GAN based on the quality of synthesized images. Earlier, GAN was being evaluated manually by visual examination of synthesized samples by the researchers or the practitioners. The manual evaluation of the GAN models suffer from the limitations of being biased and having a limit for review by human eyes within a specified time period. The GAN models should be

D Dimensional Noise Vector
Generator Network
Predicted Labels
Fake Images
Discriminator Network
Real Images

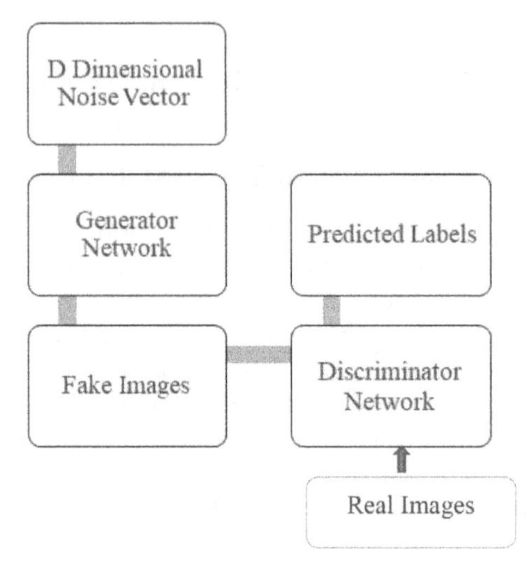

FIGURE 4.5
The Generative Adversarial Network.

Models that have high discrimination ability
Models that are sensitive to overfitting and generate diverse samples
Models that have well defined lower and upper bounds
Models that are sensitive to image distortions and transformations i.e. scoring not impacted
Is compliant with human perception and judgement
Low computational complexity

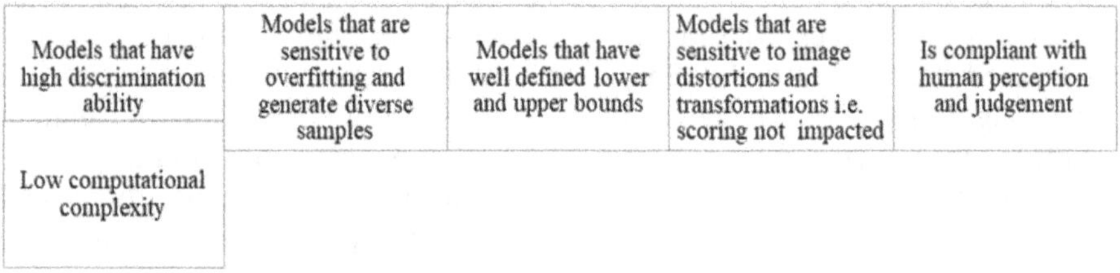

FIGURE 4.6
Criteria of a Good Evaluation Measure for GAN.

trained systematically across the cycles, and the current state of the generator should be saved for evaluation based on the images it synthesized. For an evaluation measure to be robust the necessary conditions should be met (Brownlee, 2019) and this has been shown in Figure 4.6.

There are 24 quantitative evaluation measures and 7 qualitative, of which the most frequently used Quantitative Measures are Inception Score and the Frechet Inception Distance.

The Qualitative Measure most frequently used is the Nearest Neighbor, which is used qualitatively to summarize generated images [11]. Table 4.2 below presents the popular evaluation measure to assess the futuristic framework across image quality and diversity.

Generative Adversarial Networks (GANs) have been largely in use in modern times to make visualizations that affirm the current maturity of the disease and predict the progression of the same in the near future. This chapter, while focusing on computer aided detection and diagnosis of fatal

TABLE 4.2

Evaluation Measures of GAN

Evaluation Measure	Type	Description	Calculation
Inception Score	Quantitative	Inception score is an evaluation measure that removes the subjective human evaluation of images and considers two criteria, i.e., **Quality and Diversity** of an image. The min score of the criteria is 1 and the maximum depends on the number of classes. **Conditional Probability** takes into consideration quality of the image. **Marginal Probability** considers the variety.	KLD, i.e., Kullback-Leibler Divergence between the conditional and marginal probability is given by **KL=(Conditional || Marginal) Conditional label distribution** for meaningful objects = p(n—m) that have low entropy. Large probabilities tend to suffer from information scarcity than small probabilities. Entropy is denoted as $Entropy = -\Sigma(p_i \times log(p_i))$ and **Marginal integral** is set to $p(n \mid m = G(z))dz$. Average of the KL divergence for all generated images is given by $= exp(ExKL(p(n \mid m) \mid\mid p(n)))$
Frechet Inception Distance	Quantitative	The statistical comparison between the generated vis-a-vis real samples make FID better than IS score. The output layer has 2,048 activations, from which a 2,048 feature vector is then predicted for a collection of real images.	FID = The FID score is then calculated using $d_2 = \mid\mid \mu_1 - \mu_2 \mid\mid^2 + Tr(M_1 + M_2 - 2 * (M_1 * M_2)^2)$ where d is distance, μ is featurewise mean, M_1 and M_2 are covariance matrix, Tr = the summation of the diagonal elements of the square matrix.
Nearest Neighbor	Qualitative	Is used to detect overfitting, but Nearest neighbors are used to ascertain the Euclidean distance which is extremely erogenous to small perceptual perturbations that can be alleviated by identifying more than one nearest neighbor.	

diseases at their inception using the machine learning applications, will also shed adequate light on the high level of precision achieved by the algorithms in contrast to the manual detection of terminal diseases that has challenged the scientists for a long period of time. Initially, the generator module of GAN continues to generate false images, all of which are identified by the discriminator but, with increasing number of rejections, the generator is able to learn to improve on its accuracy. More formally, given M and N where M is the set of data instances and N the set of labels:

- **Generative models** capture the joint probability of the instances and labels that is denoted by $p(M, N)$, or just $p(M)$ in absence of the labels. The generative models that predict the next word in sequence associate a probability of occurrence to the words under consideration.
- **Discriminative models** on the other hand capture the conditional probability $p(N\ M)$. But the discriminative model is only concerned with associating a label to the instance of data under consideration.

4.5.3 Case Study – Application of Generative Adversarial Network – CAD(x) Prediction of Congestive Heart Failure by GVR Creation and Usage by Neural Net

One of researches conducted in 2018 was to predict heart failure using Generative Adversarial Network, where the neural net was trained to reveal the image features like cardiomegaly, pleural effusion and airspace opacity. This research was carried out under the segment of thoracic imaging. [3]

4.5.3.1 Review of the Method

A total of 100,000-plus chest radiographs of patients were taken into consideration from year 2007 to 2016 and separated into a labeled (with B-type natriuretic peptide [BNP] as a marker of Congestive Heart Failure) and unlabeled data set. Training of the generator happened on the unlabeled data set, and the labeled data was used for training the neural network to estimate BNP, which is considered a valid marker of CHF. The resultant model was used to envision how a chest radiograph having high BNP would appear without the disease. An over-fitted model to be used for comparative evaluation was developed, and the Generative Visual Rationale was created.

A Generative Visual Rationale, otherwise known as GVR, was created, as shown in Figure 4.7, by encrypting the original image into a large vector (100 dimension) and permutations carried until the image was freed. The primary and reversed vectors were then decrypted by the generator to categorize the "diseased" synthetic and "healthy" synthetic images. The difference (that is, inclusion and exclusion of the disease) was superjacent over the primary image to produce the GVR, with the extracted density in orange and the added density in purple. The Generative Visual Rationale fundamentally was used to substantiate the change in the appearance of the chest image with respect to the stipulation that the disease did not predominate 100 GVRs using the accurately trained model, which, along with the over-fitted model

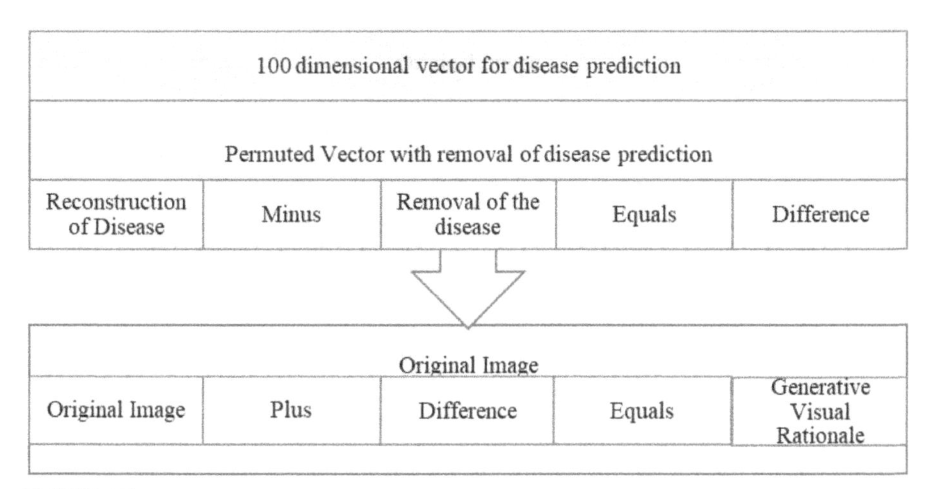

FIGURE 4.7
Creation of a Generative Visual Rationale.

was evaluated by two professionals bearing the desired expertise for features of congestive heart failure. Area under the receiver operating characteristic curve (AUC-ROC), *k* coefficient, and mixed-effects logistic regression were considered for statistical evaluation and analyses.

4.5.3.2 Review of Results

When evaluated, the Generative Visual Rationale disclosed that the model that was trained with precision, using the radiographic image features, predicted elevated BNP (B-type natriuretic peptide) as the reason for congestive heart failure more frequently than the over-fitted model. The radiographic image features that were identified and used subsequently for prediction were cardiomegaly, pleural effusions and spherical opacity.

4.5.3.3 Conclusion

Characteristics of congestive heart failure based on chest radiographs interpreted by neural networks can be found out using the Generative Visual Rationales (GVRs), sanctioning the identifying of bias and over fitted models.

4.5.3.4 Inferences and Deduction for Patient Care

Generative Visual Rationales can find out the features of the images from congestive heart failure learned by neural networks that lead to increase in BNP. Radiologists can then investigate them to uncover obscure biases, assuring riskless utilization of deep learning methodologies.

4.6 Computer Aided Diagnosis and Research Progression

Medical imaging nowadays makes provision for qualitative, diagnostic and also quantifiable information on the severity of the ailment, as well as ascertains biomarkers of diagnosis and response to treatment [12]. Computer aided diagnosis systems are evolving that provide extensive support to the decision-making process. With current advancements of the data driven methodologies, the aggregation of data-driven and conventional model-based approaches would get over some possible obstacles such as in generalizability, explain-ability and data efficiency, and better the execution of utilities such as segmentation or reconstruction of the images with improvised resolution. In the present-day health-care model, the image acquirement to rebuilding, analysis and evaluation, rendition and diagnosis is a sequential process, whereas in future it is perceived as an end-to-end pipeline [13] as shown in Figure 4.8.

4.6.1 Comparative Study of Generative versus Discriminative Algorithms

Generative and Discriminative models are primarily machine learning models some examples being the Logistic Regression, Support Vector Machine known to be of the discriminative segment, while Naive Bayes, Bayesian Networks and Hidden Markov models are among the generative ones. Both together constitute the probabilistic graphical models that act as a robust framework for encrypting probability distributions over joint distributions on a sizeable random variable set that interact with each other [14].

4.6.1.1 Model Structures

A mail classification problem to distinguish between the red spams, which are dangerous vis-a-vis the gray spams, can be considered as an example

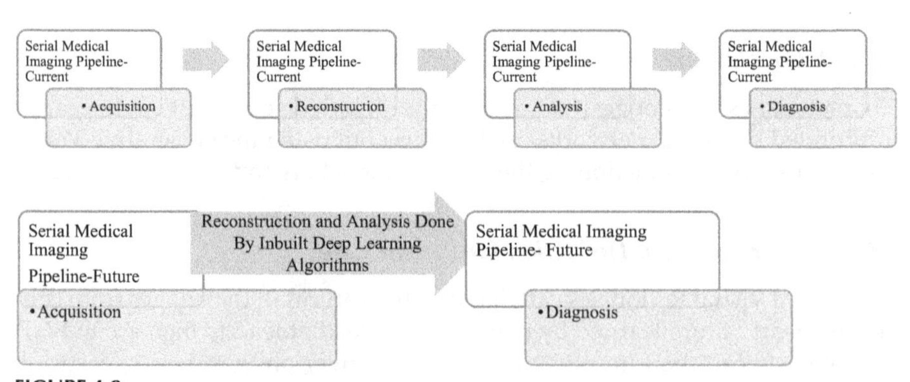

FIGURE 4.8
Serial and End-to-end Imaging Pipeline [13].

while differentiating between the above models. So a model can be created of the form as follows:

$$R = r, \text{ and features } S = s1, s2, \ldots s_m \text{ and can be as}$$
$$P(R, S) = P(R, s1, s2, \ldots s_m).$$

The ultimate objective is to estimate the probability of dangerous spams $P(R = 1\ S)$. Both generative and discriminative models can solve the above problem.

Conditional Probability can be computed by estimating prior $P(R)$ and likelihood of $P(R \mid S)$ from the training set and use Bayes rule to compute the posterior $P(R \mid S)$.

$$P\ osterior = Prior * Likelihood/Evidence \tag{1.1}$$

$$P(R \mid S) = P(R) * P(R \mid S)/P(S) \tag{1.2}$$

Discriminative models on the other hand evaluate parameters of $P(R\ S)$ directly from training data whereas Generative models infer $P(R)$ and then $P(S\ R)$ and move on to find $P(R\ S)$.

For generative models as Naive Bayes, Posterior Distribution is as follows:

$$P(R = 1 \mid S) = P(r = 1)P(s1 \mid r = 1)P(s2 \mid r = 1)P(s3 \mid r = 1)\ldots(sn \mid r = 1)/P(S)$$

For discriminative models as in Logistic Regression, the posterior distribution takes the form as:

$$P(R = 1 \mid S, a) = 1/\left(1 + exp + \sum_{a_i \times s_i}\right) \text{for } I = 1 \text{ to } S \tag{1.3}$$

As presented in Table 4.3 there are some advantages and disadvantages of the generative vis-a-vis the discriminative algorithm. While discriminative algorithms can render more accuracy, the area of coverage of generative algorithms from an application perspective is broader than discriminative models. Few of the prominent and significant researches that incorporate generative and discriminative models are cited in the form of examples below in Table 4.4.

4.6.1.2 Usage of Machine Learning and Deep Learning Algorithms in Computer Aided Diagnosis (Cad(x))

Machine learning conceptualization have been used rigorously in recent times for automated clinical analysis using the approaches as follows: semantic imaging and intelligent imaging.

TABLE 4.3

Comparison of Generative versus Discriminative Algorithms

Parameters	Generative	Discriminative
Accuracy	Less accurate as algorithm might doublecount any evidence	More accurate as α is either a 0 or 1
Missing data	Compliant	Not Compliant
Performance	Less data to train because of stronger bias	More data requisition for greater accuracy
Application	Classification, Sampling, Learning	Classification only

TABLE 4.4

Studies Conducted Using Generative and Discriminative Model

Year	Problem Statement	Result and Discussion
2016	Lung CT Analysis using both models [15]	Restricted Boltzmann machine (RBM) classification can be used to achieve the accuracy of the descriptive class that was better or closer to the findings using a set of predefined features. Incorporating discriminatory label and learning information into the standard classification technique helped produce filters that enable improvement in performance both in pure discriminatory learning and in combination yielding better results. Results showed that the random filters did very well in the tests. With large number of filters, convolution with random filters can provide useful features for partition training. Random filters being a practical foundation allows to differentiate the contribution of convolutional art to that of the learning feature algorithm.
2019	Micro calcification detection in breast mammograms using variation of both models [16]	Proposition of a new model that tackles the micro-calcification detection in mammogram images that are very small and scarce by proper usage of discriminative learning. Proposition of an Anomaly Separation Network (ASN) model to exclude proposals, and then train the differentiation network as a False Positive Reduction (FPR) model. An all inclusive convolutional encoder-decoder network is used to study the rebuild and suggests a t-test task to train the network in a controlled manner. This on examination of public and internal databases shows that this model exceeds previous technological approaches with limitation of handling the μC's.
2020	Verification of Deep Network Model [17]	Proposes to improvise on the accuracy of the abnormality detection by forecast verifications using deep D and G models. This is achieved by training a conditional verifier network p(r—s) as an approximation to the inverse posterior distribution. Deep-Verifier Networks (DVNs) achieve good accuracy on benchmark OOD discovery and adversarial example identification tasks.

Semantic Imaging can be described as the meaningful information that can act as a value-add to the existing raw data for correct interpretation of the content of the image. Meaningful interpretation includes the following: Information that is localized, such as voxel-wise organ labels and that which is global, as bounding boxes of organs or diagnostic labels. These labels consist of information about the patient or the image itself with respect to mode of the image, the acquisition rules and the precision.

This semantic imaging helps in ensuring the target segmentation where priori knowledge or otherwise known as atlas can be used and are weighted on the global, organ, and voxel level. For the global level, the rule followed is a binary weighting scheme that is applied while a continuous weighting is used in organ and voxel levels as indicated in red in Figure 4.9. Combining all the three weights it is possible to obtain spatially weighted probabilistic atlases from the set of atlas labels as shown in Figure 4.7. The final target segmentation is obtained by combining the defined spatial priors with a subject-specific intensity model in a graph-cuts based optimization step [18]. With respect to training and test images of lesions or tumors, specifically of the brain and characterized by heterogeneous appearances pertaining to locations, frequencies, shapes and extents. Machine learning techniques in those cases require to be effectual to create generalizations from the training data.

Fully 3D CNN have been deployed for brain lesion segmentation which has yielded excellent results taking into account patient data constituting of traumatic brain injuries, brain tumors, and stroke [19].

Figure 4.10 below sketches the network architecture where intermediate layers represent the brain image set and the content provided during training are multi-modal MRI's with related lesion maps. New imaging bio-markers could be revealed by such intermediaries that render accurate clinical information for assessment of critical diseases. Intermediaries in the network automatically discover the topmost attributes such as spatial positioning, alteration of gray and white matter and the ventricles. They provide valuable insights and such type of imaging techniques are known as **intelligent imaging techniques**.

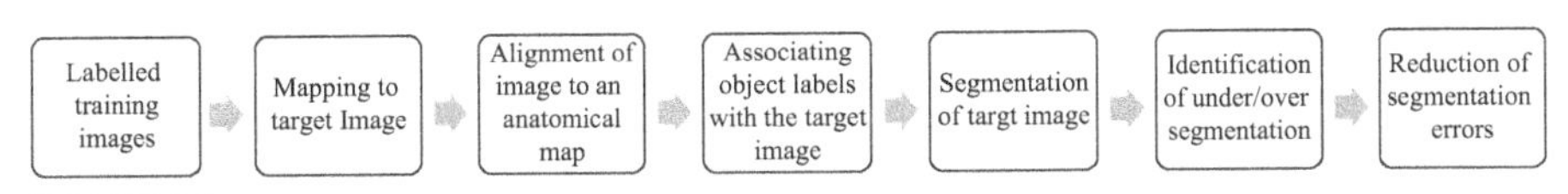

FIGURE 4.9
Usage of Atlas for Target Segmentation.

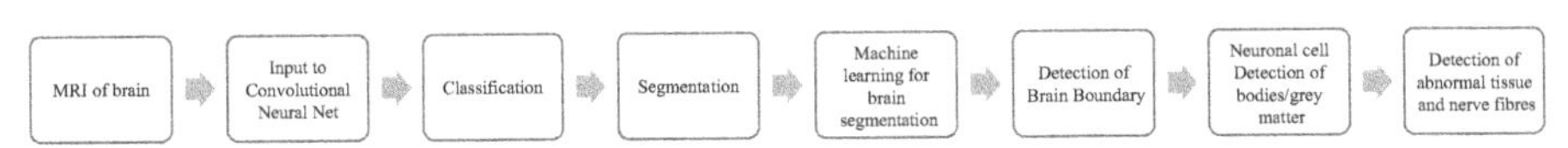

FIGURE 4.10
Brain Lesion Segmentation with DCNN.

There exist numerous deep learning applications for medical imaging which aid the clinical radiologists across various segments. They are radiomics, radiogenomics, neuro imaging, neuro radiology, brain segmentation, stroke imaging, neuro-psychiatric disorder, breast cancer, chest imaging, imaging in oncology, medical ultrasound and so forth [20]. The following Table 4.5 takes into consideration the progression along the above segments and discusses how deep learning algorithms have helped in achieving the desired levels of precision and accuracy.

TABLE 4.5

Literature Study of Usage of AI/ML Techniques in CADx

Year	AreaSegment	Authors	Result and Discussion
2014	Neuro imaging	Plis *et al.* [21]	The depth of the Deep Belief Network (DBN) is very helpful in increasing group divisions. DBN's exude resilience. DBN in conjunction with the new way of mapping can reveal hidden relationships in data.
2017	Medical ImagingReview	Tajbakhsh & Suzuki [22]	Discussion-Overview of the progression in the (1) machine learning domain pre and post the introduction of Deep Learning techniques (2) the capabilities of Deep Learning, (3) the major deep-learning models: MTANN and CNN, (4) comparative study of the two models, and (5) their contribution to the
2017	Stroke Management	Feng *et al.* [23]	Evolution of a data driven strategy for managing stroke and facilitation of prediction.
2018	Neuroradiology	Zaharchuk *et al.* [24]	Presents a summary of the recent and prospective clinical applications by emphasizing how they can change future of neuro-radiology practice. Required support from the neuro-radiology researchers will substantiate the utilization of the great power of the said novel approach.
2018	Lung and Radiomics	Hosny *et al.* [25]	The areas inside and above the tumor – chiefly the tumor-stroma interfaces are engaged in significant contributions to predict, thus elaborating on the pattern of the tissues surrounding the tumor in patient's which is chiefly facilitated by the Deep Learning.
2018	Radiogenomics	Napel *et al.* [26]	With growth of radiomics technology Deep Learning, is capable of detecting sub-tumor regions with specific constituents of cancer cell phenotypes and genotypes. These provide robust alternatives for detecting and analyzing the staging, treatment followed by monitoring the reaction.

TABLE 4.5 (Continued)

Literature Study of Usage of AI/ML Techniques in CADx

Year	AreaSegment	Authors	Result and Discussion
2019	Neuropsychiatry	Durstewitz *et al.* [27]	NN-based algorithms are capable of ingraining semantically powered computational models of brain behavior into a statistical machine learning framework and extract deeper insights into the brain dysfunction along neural and behavioral aspect.
2019	Heart	Li *et al.* [28]	Deep learning algorithms exhibited improvised accuracy, sensitivity, and specificity in identifying and classifying pulmonary nodules through CT scans that were not from the LIDCIDRI database. Discussion-No agreeable benchmark for inclusion of deep learning into the work-flow of clinical radiology for pulmonary nodules.
2019	Medical Ultrasound	Liu *et al.* [29]	Deep learning's major performance improvement greatly depends on largely training sample datasets. However, compared with the large and publicly available datasets in other areas, the current public availability of datasets in the US medical field is still limited.
2020	Chest – Thoracic CT	Halder *et al.* [30]	Visitation of earlier work leading to increase in 5-year survival rate, which at present shows that only 10–15% may be achieved. Different algorithms proposed can significantly contribute to nodule characterization based on the growth rate, that can lead to early detection of cancer and its diagnosis.

4.6.1.3 Emergence of GAN and Its Applications

Data scientists and deep learning enthusiasts use this state-of-the-art framework to perform plausible generation of photo-realistic images, change facial expression alterations, computer game simulations, visuals and so forth. Specific applications of GAN that are in common use by the industry are depicted in Figure 4.11.

GANs address the concern of "adversarial attacks" by generating false items and training the model to identify the fakes. The prime application areas of GAN are portrayed in Table 4.6.

The succeeding section will highlight the progression of computer aided diagnosis by implementing adversarial networks and further will also have an elaboration on the studies being conducted using Generative Adversarial Networks across multiple parameters. That can help in analyzing the relevant advancements in the field of computer aided medical diagnosis and emerging precision in performance. This can empower the radiologists and other clinical professionals to ensure robust and smart health-care systems.

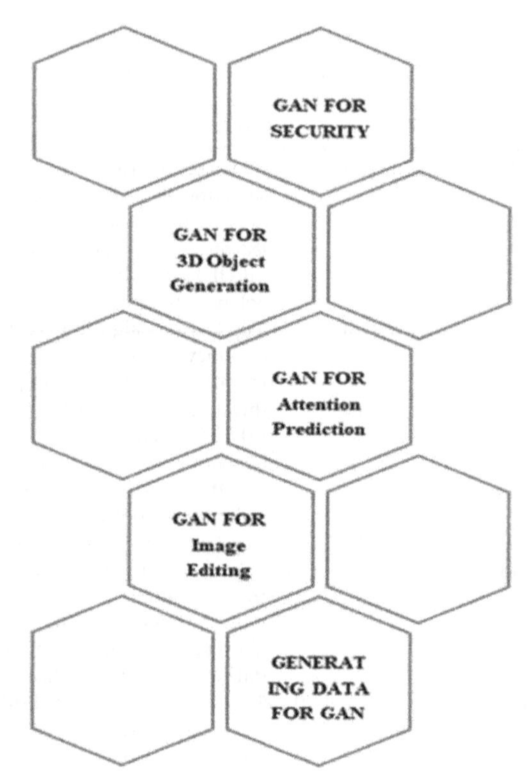

FIGURE 4.11
Applications of GAN.

TABLE 4.6
GAN Applications Other than CAMD

Security	Data Generation	Attention Prediction	3D Object Generation
GANs address the concern of "adversarial attacks" by generating fake items and training the model to identify the fakes.	Here training data is needed to model supervised learning algorithms for example healthcare.	For gaming experiences designers can focus on enhancing the features and make it more engaging.	GANs can yield 3D models by selecting from uniform noise distribution and add information of a class to both generator and discriminator model and construct a new network to create 3D conditional GAN.

4.6.1.4 *Usage of GAN in Computer Aided Diagnosis and the Stage of Maturity*

The stage of maturity as attained by Generative Adversarial Network in the segment of Image Analysis, Modality, Feature Attribution, Diagnostic Decisions and Performance Improvement through Data Augmentation is discussed in Table 4.7.

Generative models are classified as explicit and implicit. The explicit model is based on the model likelihood function, whereas the implicit generative models use a sampling technique for generation of data. Some examples of explicit models like Pixel CNN are very powerful decoders and auto encodes the images. The implicit generative models are the generative adversarial

TABLE 4.7

Literature Study of Usage of AI/ML Techniques in CADx

Segment	Stage of Maturity
Medical Image Analysis-Image translation achieved by GAN's.	GAN's application in the field of medical imaging has seen improvement with specific setups but is not uniformly seamless and needs to be further validated across categories and distribution of images.
Medical Image Analysis-Image superresolution using progressive generative adversarial networks.	Multistage P-GAN in many instances have outperformed competing methods and baseline GANs but validation needs to be done by taking into consideration PET, CT and MRI scans.
Image Modality-Generative Adversarial Networks (GAN's) for Noise Reduction in Low-Dose CT.	CNN's quality has improved by subsequent training with adversarial network to yield images with a modality that is analogous to cited routine-dose CT images. This has helped in steering the improvement in performance by ensuring reduction in noise with better resolution.
Feature Attribution Variant of GAN termed as WGAN's usage for visual feature attribution.	Wasserstein Generative Adversarial Networks (WGAN), performs considerably finer for ocular attribution on synthetic dataset.
Computer Aided Medical Diagnosis Visual Turing Test using Deep Convolutional GAN's.	DC-GAN's have the potential to ameliorate diagnostic decisions by excavating highly discriminative imaging attributes and can generate realistic samples for training deep networks making use of big data 'with reference to identification of malignant and benign cells.
Computer Aided Detection – Through Data Augmentation by GAN	GAN's have become a workable technique of data augmentation for nodule discovery and are segments that accrue for potential research in the CADe. They have the potential to generate more training data.

networks whose usage and relevance to image synthesizing is of significant value today. While explicit models are trained by maximizing the likelihood, the implicit ones approximate a data distribution, using a parameterized model distribution. Here the generator G is trained to produce an image from a noise vector that is in proximity to the true data distribution, whereas the discriminator D differentiates between the synthesized and the original images. This chapter having dealt with computer aided detection, diagnosis and the role of AI in assisting the medical professionals in taking critical clinical decisions, now aims at presenting the application of GAN and its variants, like PGAN, AnoGAN, WGAN, and STAR GAN's contribution in the disease diagnosis specifically by augmenting, synthesizing, analyzing the images along with anomaly detection. This along with the diverse measures of performance-like precision, recall, FIndex, Dice Coefficient, Hausdorff Peak to Signal Noise Ratio, Mean Absolute Error, Sensitivity, Specificity, AUC-ROC, Structured Similarity Index, KL Divergence Score will also provide insight into the most commonly used metrics required to evaluate the robustness of GAN and also the diagnostic system and provide detailed in-depth insight into the applicability of GAN in CAD. Hence a detailed review has been conducted and presented in Table 4.8.

4.7 Generative Adversarial Network and Its Contribution to Computer Aided Diagnosis

4.7.1 Discussion and Conclusion

GAN's capability to model high-dimensional data, handling missing data, and making provisions for multiple plausible answers in the segment of image synthesis and translation, has culminated in frequent usage of this technique in computer aided diagnosis. Computer aided diagnosis/detection is interdisciplinary and is the confluence of pathology, radiology, artificial intelligence and machine learning. Hence it has seen the contribution of the state-of-the-art architecture like GAN. CAD's robustness is measured using Sensitivity, Specificity and Absolute Detection Rate whereas the most standard evaluation measure of GAN is the inception score. Sensitivity and Specificity of the Inception scores are measured to understand the robustness of GAN. In addition, the classification algorithms that are used especially for diagnosis consist of Naive Bayesian Classifier (NBC), Support Vector Machine (SVM), Principal Component Analysis (PCA) and Artificial Neural Network (ANN) using which every Region of Interest (ROI) is analyzed. It is said that with AI adoption, the best results are achieved when the disease detection happens first manually and then with CAD. As a result, less percentage change is exuded in disease detection with CAD intervention

TABLE 4.8

Application of GAN in Computer Aided Diagnosis (Research Review)

Sl. No.	Year	Authors	Objective	Research Area	Region of Interest	GAN Type and Model	Performance Parameters	Results Discussion	Citation
3	2019	Siddiquee *et.al.* [32]	FP GAN-Supervising samedomain and regularizing cross domain translation, the initial through conditional identity loss and the later through revised adversarial, domain classification, and cycle consistency loss	Medical Imaging	Image translation	FP GAN for cross domain translation and comparing with STAR GAN	Derivation of a FP GAN for an ailment discovery and determining the location using image-level annotation based on FP translation learning. Betterment over STAR GAN	The precision and accuracy of generated images by FP GAN is in close propinquity to the original images, emphasizing the need and strength of FP translational – learning in cross-domain translation. Accuracy FP GAN -92.31 STAR GAN -90.82%.	9
4	2017	Schlegl *et.al.* [33]	Proposing AnoGAN, a DCGAN,to learn multiple normal anatomical variations that is associated by a new anomaly scoring scheme based on image to latent space mapping.	Retinopathy	Retinal Anomaly Detection	Performance assessment for detecting the Anomaly. The GANR, the a CAE and the AnoGAN on image-level labels.	ePrecision Recall Sensitivity Specificity AUC	AnoGAN out performed others in precision, recall, sensitivity and specificity and AUC the values of which are as follows: 0.8834 0.7277 0.7279 0.8928 0.89	611

(continued)

TABLE 4.8 (Continued)

Application of GAN in Computer Aided Diagnosis (Research Review)

Sl. No.	Year	Authors	Objective	Research Area	Region of Interest	GAN Type and Model	Performance Parameters	Results Discussion	Citation
5	2019	Yu *et al.* [34]	Enhancement in the quality of the image synthesis	Medical Imaging Synthesis	Retinal Image Synthesis	Multiple-channels multiple landmarks (MCML) Cycle GAN architecture	SSIM and PSNR(Structural Similarity Index(SI) and Peak to Signal Noise Ratio(PSNR)	MCML out-performs the single vessel-based methods for each architecture of GAN's. Fusion with multichannel attains 94% accuracy i.e. structural similarity index	5
6	2018	Pan *et.al.* [35]	2 stage DL framework for brain ailment categorization with MRI and PET data. Image Synthesis by 3D-cGAN and implementation of Landmark based multimodal multi-instance learning	Medical Image Synthesis	MRI/PET Image Synthesis for Alzheimer's disease	Development of a deep convolutional multi-instance neural network for AD diagnosis and conversion and forecast of MCI	Accuracy (ACC), sensitivity (SEN), specificity (SPE), F1 - Score (F1 S), the area under receiver operating characteristic (AUCROC) and Matthews correlation coefficient (MCC)	92.50 89.94 94.53 91.37 84.78 95.89 79.06 55.26 82.85 40.86 30.13 75.84 LM3IL outperforms others	15

7	2020	Tang *et al.* [36]	Synthesizing CT realistic images from non-generic lymph node masks using Data augmentation approach	Medical Imaging	Lymph node Segmentation	pix2pix GAN model for image generation robust u net model for learning	DICE Score	An increase in the performance with the Dice score increased about 2.2% (from 80.3% to 82.5%) for realistic CT images and the sectionalization of the lymph node	15
8	2019	Chen *et al.* [37]	Through Adversarial learning, better the quality of medical image segmentation and create a novel segment or network using a receptive field block (RFB) module for precise feature extraction.	Medical Data Analysis	Prostrate Image Analysis and Synthesis	GAN impregnated with Receptor Field Block	Quantitative comparison with other segmentation methods in Dice similarity coefficient (DSC) and (HD) Hausdorff distance	For the proposed method the DSC = 88.27 HD = 8.0 and this method outperformed others	2
9	2018	Shin *et al.* [38]	Generation of artificial abnormal MRI images of brain tumors by training a GAN using two brain MRI datasets that are available publicly. Using the artificially generated in the form of extended data sets for enhanced performance	Medical Image Synthesis	Brain tumour segmentation using Data Augmentation and anomymization	Translation GAN with and without augmentation (Removal of crop, rotation and elastic deformation	Dice score evaluation (mean / standard deviation) translation	Improved segmentation masks using an image-to-image translation GAN.	149

(continued)

TABLE 4.8 (Continued)

Application of GAN in Computer Aided Diagnosis (Research Review)

Sl. No.	Year	Authors	Objective	Research Area	Region of Interest	GAN Type and Model	Performance Parameters	Results Discussion	Citation
10	2017	Dong *et al.* [39]	Convolutional network designed (FCN) to generate CT from a MRI.	Medical Image Synthesis	CT Imaging	Usage of a GAN with convolution network as generator with image gradient loss function and usage of adversarial training strategy using discriminator along with auto context model	Peak to Signal Noise Ratio (PSNR) and Mean Absolute Error(MAE)	3D GAN model with Auto Context model executes better than other efficient methods and can be made usable for denoising and super resolution. Proposed Model MAE (Mean and Median) 92.5 (std 13.9) 92.1 PSNR – 27.6(1.3) 27.6	302
11	2019	Li *et.al.* [40]	Multivariate Anomaly Detection GAN (MAD-GAN) is a model that is used to ascertain complex multivariate correlations among the many data streams to proctor invasion through abnormalcy identification.	Anomaly Detection	Cyber-physical-systems (CPSs)	MAD GAN with LSTM RNN and Anamoly Detector	Precision, Recall and F-Index	MAD GAN had outperformed for unbalanced data-sets with precision of 99.99 pc, recall of 99.98 and F 1 of .77	45

12	2020	Zhang *et al.* [41]	Unsupervised X-ray image segmentation and image synthesis and parsing between annotated DRRs and unannotated X-rays.	Medical Imaging	X-ray image synthesis and segmentation	GAN's that are task driven constitute of varied cycleGAN substructure for pixel-to-pixel translation between DRRs and X-ray images. It implements the pretrained DI2I to acquire deep supervision and enforces agreeable performance on partition-	Dice Coefficient	Accuracy of 86 pc in contrast to supervised training with a dice coefficient of 89 pc.	6

than the percentage increase in the recall rate. Generative and discriminative models are primarily machine learning models, some examples being the Logistic Regression and SVM known to be of the discriminative type, while Naive Bayes, Bayesian Networks and Hidden Markov models are among the generative ones. The comparison and the contrast of the Generative and the Discriminative Models are generally done based on Accuracy, Missing Data, Performance and Applications. Machine learning approaches have been used rigorously in recent times for automated clinical analysis using the approaches as follows: Semantic imaging and intelligent imaging that focuses on information localization and retrieval of the same such as voxel-wise organ labels and accessing the bounding boxes of organs that are considered to be global in category. In addition, the global categories of information being the diagnostic labels such as information about the patient or the image itself with respect to modality and quality. There exist numerous applications of deep learning for medical imaging which aid the clinical radiologists specifically in the segments of radiomics, radiogenomics, neuro imaging and radiology, brain segmentation and imaging, neuro-psychiatric disorder, breast carcinoma, chest tomography, imaging in oncology and medical ultrasonography. 3D CNN have been deployed for brain lesion segmentation which has yielded excellent results taking into consideration multi-modal data from patients and so forth. Deep learning algorithms, when implemented for diagnosing and classifying pulmonary nodules on CT scans, exuded a high level of accuracy, sensitivity and specificity. Wasserstein Generative Adversarial Networks (WGAN), on the other hand, performs substantially better than the progressive algorithms for visual attribution on synthetic dataset. DC-GANs can improvise on the decision-making by mining highly discriminative imaging features and can generate realistic samples for training deep networks, making use of big data. GANs can accurately detect lung nodules using the technique of data augmentation and can be considered to be an area having potential for research. The Deep Belief Network, in conjunction with a new way of mapping, can reveal hidden relationships in medical image data. NN-based algorithms, on the other hand, can embed semantically explainable machine models of brain kinetics or conduct into a statistical machine learning context. In case of GAN and its variants applicability in the field of computer aided diagnosis, it is found that WGAN enables fine grained classification with greater accuracy, precision and recall up to 95 percent in nodule detection, and is able to train on positive data sets, whereas the Dual GAN crafted using a two-stage approach synthesizes images with an FI accuracy closer to 90 percent. The type of Generative Adversarial Network AnoGAN used for anomaly detection exudes a precision, recall, sensitivity and specificity value which is more than 85 percent for the majority of the assessment measures. For image translation the Fixed Point GAN has reached an accuracy of 92 percent and quality of generated images are much closer to the original ones. The task-driven GAN, on the other hand, with its deep supervising capabilities ensures consistent image segmentation. Some GAN frameworks have also achieved a dice coefficient of 0.837 and .832 for STARE and DRIVE data set respectively, which is state-of-the-art performance and promises of opportunities in the segment of diagnosis. Adversarial networks now exude great commitment in the segment of CAD(x) and results received can range from reliability and efficiency to lowering costs for clinics and hospitals and at the same time provide the needed support to the clinicians and radiologists to make the health-care system smarter and better.

4.8 Future Scope

Generative Adversarial Networks in the field of medical imaging and analysis have experienced huge research potential. Though there are multiple challenges connected to the inclusion of GAN in clinical environments, still the techniques exhibit superiority that is too important to abandon, owing to numerous research articles published in premium journals in the segment of medical imaging and analysis. Further to this, with extensive use of technology, the practitioners can gain experience to classify problems based on the solution strategies, that is, using the best possible approach, using deep learning approaches in totality or using the methodologies in combination. GANs and other deep learning techniques' potential can be leveraged, to make more robust the technological inclination of medical practitioners for whom the usage of high-end software for clinical diagnosis would become a second habit and help in transformation to a newfound medical paradigm that is prognostic, prophylactic, individualized and participatory in nature.

References

[1] Yiming Gao, Krzysztof J. Geras, & Alana A. Lewin. New frontiers: An update on computer-aided diagnosis for breast imaging in the age of artificial intelligence. *American Journal of Roentgenology*, 212(2): 300–307, 2019.

[2] Bradley J. Erickson & Brian Bartholmai. Computer-aided detection and diagnosis at the start of the third millennium. *Journal of Digital Imaging: The Official Journal of the Society for Computer Applications in Radiology*, 15: 59–68, 2002.

[3] Jarrel C. Y. Seah, Jennifer S. N. Tang, Andy Kitchen, Frank Gaillard, & Andrew F. Dixon. Chest radiographs in congestive heart failure: Visualizing neural network learning. *Radiology*, 290(2): 514–522, 2019.

[4] Ronald A Castellin. Computer aided detection (cad): an overview. *Cancer Imaging*, 5(1): 17–19, 2005.

[5] Constance D. Lehman, Robert D. Wellman, Diana S. M. Buist, Karla Kerlikowske, Anna N. A. Tosteson, & Diana L. Miglioretti. Diagnostic accuracy of digital screening mammography with and without computer-aided detection. *JAMA Internal Medicine*, 175(11): 1828–1837, Nov. 2015.

[6] Natalia Pirouzbakht & J. Mejia. *Algorithm for the detection of breast cancer in digital mammograms using deep learning*. 2017.

[7] Thijs Kooi, Geert Litjens, Bram Ginneken, Albert Gubern-Meťrida, Clara Saťnchez, Ritse Mann, Gerard Heeten, & Nico Karssemeijer. Large scale deep learning for computer aided detection of mammographic lesions. *Medical Image Analysis*, 35: 303–312, 08 2016.

[8] Chunli Qin, Demin Yao, Yonghong Shi, & Zhijian Song. Computer-aided detection in chest radiography based on artificial intelligence: a survey. *Bio-Medical Engineering Online*, 17(113), 2018.

[9] Hamido Fujita & Dalibor Cimr. Computer aided detection for fibrillations and flutters using deep convolutional neural network. *Information Sciences*, 486, 02 2019.

[10] Masashi Misawa, Shin ei Kudo, Yuichi Mori, Kinichi Hotta, Kazuo Ohtsuka, Takahisa Matsuda, Shoichi Saito, Toyoki Kudo, Toshiyuki Baba, Fumio Ishida, Hayato Itoh, & Masahiro Oda Kensaku Mori. Development of a computer-aided detection system for colonoscopy and a publicly accessible large colonoscopy video database. *Gastrointestinal Endoscopy*, 7 2020.

[11] Ali Borji. Pros and cons of GAN evaluation measures. 10.13140/RG.2.2.16789.42720, 2018.

[12] Marcel Koenigkam Santos, José Raniery Ferreira Júnior, Danilo Tadao Wada, Ariane Priscilla Magalhães Tenório, Marcello Henrique Nogueira Barbosa, & Paulo Mazzoncini de Azevedo Marques. Artificial intelligence, machine learning, computer-aided diagnosis, and radiomics: advances in imaging towards to precision medicine. *Radiol Bras*, 52(6): 387–396, 2019.

[13] D. Rueckert & J. A. Schnabel. Model-based and data-driven strategies in medical image computing. *Proceedings of the IEEE*, 108(1): 110–124, 2020.

[14] Siwei Xu. *Generative vs. discriminative probabilistic graphical models*, 04 2019.

[15] Gijs van Tulder & Marleen de Bruijne. Combining generative and discriminative representation learning for lung CT analysis with convolutional restricted Boltzmann machines. *IEEE Transactions on Medical Imaging*, 35: 1–1, 02 2016.

[16] F. Zhang, L. Luo, X. Sun, Z. Zhou, X. Li, Y. Yu, & Y. Wang. Cascaded generative and discriminative learning for microcalcification detection in breast mammograms. In *2019 IEEE/CVF Conference on Computer Vision and Pattern Recognition (CVPR)*, pp. 12570–12578, 2019.

[17] Tong Che, Xiaofeng Liu, Site Li, Yubin Ge, Ruixiang Zhang, Caiming Xiong, & Yoshua Bengio. Deep verifier networks: Verification of deep discriminative models with deep generative models, 2020.

[18] R. Wolz, C. Chu, K. Misawa, M. Fujiwara, K. Mori, & D. Rueckert. Automated abdominal multi-organ segmentation with subject-specific atlas generation. *IEEE Transactions on Medical Imaging*, 32(9): 1723–1730, 2013.

[19] Konstantinos Kamnitsas, Christian Ledig, Virginia F. J. Newcombe, Joanna P. Simpson, Andrew D. Kane, David K. Menon, Daniel Rueckert, & Ben Glocker. Efficient multiscale 3d CNN with fully connected CRF for accurate brain lesion segmentation. Computing Research Repository,abs/1603.05959, 2016.

[20] Alexander Selvikvåg Lundervold & Arvid Lundervold. An overview of deep learning in medical imaging focusing on MRI. *Zeitschrift fur medizinische Physik*, 29(2): 102–127, 2019.
[21] Sergey M. Plis, Devon R. Hjelm, Ruslan Salakhutdinov, Elena A. Allen, Henry J. Bockholt, Jeffrey D. Long, Hans J. Johnson, Jane S. Paulsen, Jessica A. Turner, & Vince D. Calhoun. Deep learning for neuroimaging: a validation study. *Frontiers in Neuroscience*, 8(229). http://dx.doi.org/10.3389/fnins.2014.00229.
[22] Nima Tajbakhsh & Kenji Suzuki. *A comparative study of modern machine learning approaches for focal lesion detection and classification in medical images: BoVW, CNN and MTANN*, pp. 31–58. 01 2018.
[23] Rui Feng, Marcus Badgeley, J. Mocco, & Eric K. Oermann. Deep learning guided stroke management: a review of clinical applications. *Journal of NeuroInterventional Surgery*, 10(4): 358–362, 2018.
[24] G. Zaharchuk, E. Gong, M. Wintermark, D. Rubin, & C. P. Langlotz. Deep learning in neuroradiology. *American Journal of Neuroradiology*, 2018.
[25] Ahmed Hosny, Chintan Parmar, Thibaud P. Coroller, Patrick Grossmann, Roman Zeleznik, Avnish Kumar, Johan Bussink, Robert J. Gillies, Raymond H. Mak, & Hugo J. W. L. Aerts. Deep learning for lung cancer prognostication: A retrospective multi-cohort radiomics study. *PLOS Medicine*, 15(11): 1–25, 11 2018.
[26] Sandy Napel, Wei Mu, Bruna V. Jardim-Perassi, Hugo J. W. L. Aerts, & Robert J. Gillies. Quantitative imaging of cancer in the postgenomic era: Radio(geno) mics, deep learning, and habitats. *Cancer*, 124(24): 4633–4649, 2018.
[27] Daniel Durstewitz, Georgia Koppe, & Andreas MeyerLindenberg. Deep neural networks in psychiatry. *Molecular Psychiatry*, 24(11): 1583–1598, 2019.
[28] Dana Li, Bolette Mikela Vilmun, Jonathan Frederik Carlsen, Elisabeth Albrecht-Beste, Carsten Ammitzb0l Lauridsen, Michael Bachmann Nielsen, & Kristoffer Lindskov Hansen. The performance of deep learning algorithms on automatic pulmonary nodule detection and classification tested on different datasets that are not derived from lidc-idri: A systematic review. *Diagnostics*, 9(4): 207, 2019.
[29] Shengfeng Liu, Yi Wang, Xin Yang, Baiying Lei, Li Liu, Shawn Xiang Li, Dong Ni, and Tianfu Wang. Deep learning in medical ultrasound analysis: A review. *Engineering*, 5(2): 261, 2019.
[30] Amitava Halder, Debangshu Dey, & Anup Sadhu. Lung nodule detection from feature engineering to deep learning in thoracic CT images: a comprehensive review. *Journal of Digital Imaging*, 33, 01 2020.
[31] John T. Guibas, Tejpal S. Virdi, & Peter S. Li. Synthetic medical images from dual generative adversarial networks, 2018.
[32] Md Mahfuzur Rahman Siddiquee, Zongwei Zhou, Nima Tajbakhsh, Ruibin Feng, Michael B. Gotway, Yoshua Bengio, & Jianming Liang. Learning fixed points in generative adversarial networks: From image-to-image translation to disease detection and localization, 2019.
[33] Thomas Schlegl, Philipp Seeböck, Sebastian M. Waldstein, Georg Langs, & Ursula Schmidt-Erfurth. f-anogan: Fast unsupervised anomaly detection with generative adversarial networks. *Medical Image Analysis*, 54: 30–44, 2019.
[34] Zekuan Yu, Qing Xiang, Jiahao Meng, Caixia Kou, Qiushi Ren, & Yanye Lu. Retinal image synthesis from multiple-landmarks input with generative adversarial networks. *BioMedical Engineering OnLine*, 18(1): 62, May 2019.

[35] Yongsheng Pan, Mingxia Liu, Chunfeng Lian, Tao Zhou, Yong Xia, & Dinggang Shen. Synthesizing missing PET from MRI with cycle-consistent generative adversarial networks for Alzheimersť Disease diagnosis. In Alejandro F. Frangi, Ju-lia A. Schnabel, Christos Davatzikos, Carlos Alberola-Lopez, & Gabor Fichtinger, editors, *Medical Image Computing and Computer Assisted Intervention*, pp. 455–463. Springer, 2018.

[36] You-Bao Tang, Sooyoun Oh, Yu-Xing Tang, Jing Xiao, & Ronald M. Summers. CT-realistic data augmentation using generative adversarial network for robust lymph node segmentation. In Kensaku Mori & Horst K. Hahn, editors, *Medical Imaging 2019: Computer-Aided Diagnosis*, volume 10950, pp. 976–981. International Society for Optics and Photonics, SPIE, 2019.

[37] Ailian Chen, Leilei Zhu, Huaijuan Zang, Zhenglong Ding, & Shu Zhan. Computer aided diagnosis and decision-making system for medical data analysis: A case study on prostate MR images. *Journal of Management Science and Engineering*, 4(4): 266–278, 2019.

[38] Hoo-Chang Shin, Neil A. Tenenholtz, Jameson K. Rogers, Christopher G. Schwarz, Matthew L. Senjem, Jeffrey L. Gunter, Katherine P. Andriole, & Mark Michalski. Medical image synthesis for data augmentation and anonymization using generative adversarial networks. In Ali Gooya, Orcun Goksel, Ipek Oguz, & Ninon Burgos, editors, *Simulation and Synthesis in Medical Imaging*, pp. 1–11. Springer, 2018.

[39] Dong Nie, Roger Trullo, Jun Lian, Caroline Petitjean, Su Ruan, Qian Wang, & Dinggang Shen. Medical image synthesis with context-aware generative adversarial networks. In Maxime Descoteaux, Lena Maier-Hein, Alfred Franz, Pierre Jannin, D. Louis Collins, & Simon Duchesne, editors, *Medical image computing and computer assisted intervention – MICCAI 2017*, pp. 417–425, Cham, 2017. Springer.

[40] Dan Li, Dacheng Chen, Baihong Jin, Lei Shi, Jonathan Goh, & See-Kiong Ng. Mad-gan: Multivariate anomaly detection for time series data with generative adversarial networks. In (eds) Igor V. Tetko, Veıra KΨurkovať, Pavel Karpov, and Fabian Theis, *Artificial Neural Networks and Machine Learning – ICANN 2019: Text and Time Series*, pp. 703–716. Springer, 2019.

[41] Yue Zhang, Shun Miao, Tommaso Mansi, & Rui Liao. Unsupervised x-ray image segmentation with task driven generative adversarial networks. *Medical Image Analysis*, 62: 101664, 2020.

5

A Critical Review of Machine Learning Techniques for Diagnosing the Corona Virus Disease (COVID-19)

Khushbu Kumari, Rik Das, Pankaj Kumar Manjhi, and Satya Narayan Singh

CONTENTS

5.1 Introduction

Current times have experienced the spread of COVID-19 as a pandemic with vast numbers of cases of infection across the globe. COVID-19 is an ongoing outbreak with worldwide influence. It often results in Severe Acute Respiratory Syndrome (SARS) and is also named as SARS-Cov-2 [1]. The preliminary symptoms of COVID 19 includes cough, fever, weariness and body pain [2], whereas at later stages the infected body faces other difficulties, including breathing problems, heart-related problems and other infections [3]. Since December 2019, the novel corona virus disease has emerged with symptoms of Acute Respiratory Distress Syndrome (ARDS) in the Wuhan city (China). Thereafter, it is continuously expanding with large community spread that has affected over two hundred countries worldwide, including China, the United States, the United Kingdom, Russia, Brazil, Spain, Italy, Peru, India, France, Germany and so on [4] [5] [6].

This disease has created major distress in public health at the international level, with large community spread. Thus, the World Health Organization announced it as an international health emergency [7].

The research community is carrying out intense exploration to offer remedies, by means of novel technological and medical methodologies, for this stringent challenge of an ongoing pandemic. The proposed technologies will be helpful for better monitoring of infected patients by close observation of related Covid-19 medical cases and with reduced human contact with infected people.

Artificial Intelligence and machine learning techniques have taken a pivotal role in controlling the spread of Covid-19 by helping in diagnosing the disease with different effective techniques, such as advanced artificial intelligence techniques coupled with automated radiology imaging techniques such as CT scans and chest X-rays, DarkNet models with YOLO(You Only Look Once), which is mainly a real-time object detection system, and so forth [8] [9] [10]. The artificial intelligence-based models are also able to identify the corona virus symptoms at an early stage and can attempt to accurately predict the mortality risk by analyzing previous data from diverse environments [11].

The main application of learning based systems in detection and diagnosis of Covid-19 epidemic are as follows:(i) possible detection of the Covid-19 infection in patients in the primary stage due to agile decision-making processes with the help of automated learning techniques; (ii) diagnosis of corona virus disease by using technologies based on medical images – for example; chest X-ray images, CT scan images and magnetic resonance imaging (MRI) images; (iii) easy monitoring of patients by using extracted phenomenal features of the corona virus disease and applying them for treatment of disease; (iv) predicting the rate of infected cases, active cases, mortality rate and discharged cases with the help of automated learning based models for keeping track of related Covid-19 cases; (v) development of vaccines with the help of advance artificial intelligence based technology; (vi) prevention and cure of disease rooted in real-time data analysis; (vii) future reappearance of such kinds of disease or the same, and so forth [12].

Since COVID-19 infected patients have faced heavy respiratory problems, the CT images of lungs are useful for understanding the level of infection. Thus, computer aided diagnosis is one of the widely emerging system used by the medical sector for dealing with image quality as well as the classification of medical images based on machine vision methods. Whereas, with the help of the learning based models, the treatment of disease is getting simpler at early stages of COVID-19 [13].

This chapter deals with the review of the diverse machine learning techniques, with all their critics, which have been developed for fighting corona virus disease in the field of medical imaging diagnosis. This research may help to analyze the existing machine learning models, with their efficiency and performance accuracy, for identification and treatment of the COVID-19 disease.

5.2 Literature Review

COVID-19 is spreading alarmingly across the world as a pandemic. For dealing with COVID-19 cases, the medical sector is widely using techniques based on the radiology images, namely chest X-rays, CT images, MRI scans and so forth. During the present battle with corona virus, it is a necessity to diagnose the disease at a much faster rate and with unprecedented accuracy. Machine learning techniques are playing a vital role in fighting corona cases with its effective learning based methods.

Convolutional neural networks (CNNs) [14] are emerging as one of the most reliable techniques for investigating COVID-19 cases with medical images such as, Computed Tomography (CT) images, chest X-rays, magnetic resonance imaging (MRI). In addition, other pre-trained models like InceptionV3, ResNet50 architecture, VGG16 and so on have also exhibited state-of-the-art performance in COVID detection and diagnosis [15]. Much research is being carried out for diagnosing corona virus disease with the help of machine learning methods and diverse classifiers such as Linear Regression, Logistic Regression, Naive Bayes classifiers, support vector machines, K-nearest neighbor and so forth [16]. These studies clearly emphasize that with the help of machine learning techniques, it is getting simpler to diagnose and monitor corona virus disease in effective manner.

5.3 Machine Learning Techniques for Diagnosis of Corona Virus Disease through Medical Images

Presently, machine learning methods are extensively used for diagnosing COVID cases with the help of radiological imaging techniques. The amalgamation of traditional radiological imaging techniques with machine learning methods are giving better results with improved classification performance in detection of COVID cases. A lot of research has already been done in the field of computer aided medical diagnosis, which continuously gives valuable insights for diagnosing COVID cases and fighting the disease.

A recent deep learning based new proposition named COVID-Net [17] is designed for diagnosing corona virus disease by using chest X-ray images at an earlier phase. COVID-Net focuses on predicting the intense intimation regarding COVID infections. The model COVID-Net uses an open-access dataset named COVIDx, which is mainly used to perform the test by comparing more than thirteen thousand normal chest X-ray images with a similar number of X-ray images from COVID patients. The proposed dataset has been fabricated for performing the classification by separating train and test dataset for detection of COVID disease. The model achieved 98.9 percent of precision for corona virus infected cases.

Research proposed [18] a Residual Network based model called CAAD (confidence-aware anomaly detection) for diagnosing corona virus disease by working with chest X-ray images. The model principally focuses on two things: in the first stage, it is segregating COVID and Non-COVID cases, whereas in the second stage, the detection of ambiguity is performed in the classified data. This research involved datasets with a binary assortment that includes a dataset named X-VIRAL, having 5,977 viral infection cases, 18,619 non-viral cases and 18,774 cases that are free from any infection, whereas in the other side X-COVID dataset, contains 106 COVID positive cases with 107 normal cases. The mentioned model has contributed towards the study of corona virus pandemic by achieving 83.61 percent precision for COVID detection.

A deep learning method based on supervised learning named DeCoVNet [19] is proposed to find the COVID infection in the human body through lung segmentation via 3D convolutional neural network and pre-trained UNet. The DeCoVNet is a 3-D convolutional neural network consisting of three blocks of network – namely, stem, residual block and fully connected layer with activation function. This model has focused to foreshow the infection inference of COVID-19 with the assistance of supervised deep learning classification algorithm. The research has used 499 CT scan images for preparing a training set and 131 CT images for testing cases with performance accuracy of 90.1 percent. However, the main objective of the model is to minimize the performance time for detection of COVID cases, and it has achieved the result with a mere 1.93 seconds for each CT scan.

Another recent technique [20] has constructed a machine learning model using U-Net++,a segmentation model based learning method for diagnosing the disease by using a total of 49,096 CT images from 51 COVID infected patients and 55 patients with other infection types. In this research, the primary focus is to reduce the convergence time for classification with the help of deep learning methods, which achieved better performance efficiency in the classification of radiological images as well as it has provided a better way to stop community spread of virus by minimizing the clinical team contact with COVID patients by applying an intelligence monitoring system for early diagnosis. The research has acquired 98.85 percent performance accuracy for screening and identification with a single CT image as well as having curtailed the performance time up to 65 percent.

A blended framework [21] of deep learning architecture named ResNet 50 and UNet++ have been used as a combined system aimed for improving classification accuracy by minimizing testing time and maximizing testing performance with the help of deep learning methods for corona virus disease detection by using CT images as a test bed. This machine learning based model has incorporated four steps: compilation of images data, labeling, preparing training data and executing the system for screening of COVID-19 detection.

COVID-ResNet [22], a pre-trained CNN with Residual Network of 50 layered architecture is proposed as a learning based model for diagnosing COVID-19 infection from radiological images. COVID-ResNet mainly aimed to increase the classification performance through minimizing the training time for COVID detection and recorded 96.23 percent of classification accuracy.

A machine learning based model named DeTraC [23] has been constructed to classify corona virus infected X-ray images by confrontation with three stages: Decompose, Transfer and Compose. The first state of the model focused on extracting important features from chest X-ray images and train it, whereas the second phase involves the decomposition process by applying optimization for elucidating the classification, and the last has dealt with sublimating the classified images. The model mainly targeted understanding abnormality among the image dataset by applying the decomposition method for classification and has achieved classification accuracy of 95.12 percent.

One more research [24] has proposed comparison of deep learning technique using three discontinuous architectures: ResNet50, InceptionV3 and the Inception-ResNetV2 model for COVID detection on dataset taken by X-ray images. This research has clearly shown that out of the three mentioned architectures, ResNet50 (a Residual Network of 50 layers) has recorded the best result. According to this research the deep learning method with ResNet50 architecture for detection of COVID cases has been securing 98 percent of performance accuracy in comparison to InceptionV3, which secures 97 percent of classification accuracy, and Inception-ResNetV2 with 87 percent of performance accuracy.

A model named BCNN (Bayesian Convolutional Neural Network) [25] has been constructed to diagnose the corona virus cases through predicting the suspected COVID-19 cases. According to this research, a trained set of deep learning classifiers have been prepared by using transfer learning methods which have given a better accuracy in predicting uncertainty.

COVIDx-Net [26], a deep learning structure, is designed for COVID case monitoring and diagnosis. The model involved different convolutional neural network architecture such as VGG19, Mobile-NetV2, Xception, Inception-ResNetV2, InceptionV3, DensNet201 and so forth for comparing the performance outcome for classification of COVID19 infected cases. The result recorded a highest accuracy of 90 percent with VGG19 and the same for DensNet201 rather than the other mentioned architecture models.

These mentioned models have achieved satisfactory performances in different manners for diagnosing COVID-19 and contributing valuable insights for the fight against the pandemic.

5.4 Discussion and Analysis

The application of COVID disease detection through deep learning methods is now becoming an emerging research domain in the field of clinical radiography. The present chapter has purposely tried to examine the automated deep learning based feature extraction techniques for diagnosing the COVID-19 cases with chest X-rays and Computed Tomography (CT) scan based on the radiological images. Chest X-ray and CT images are widely used as medical screening techniques for identification of disease as well as finding the level of infection in an individual with the help of radiological images. Hence, it is becoming important to classify those medical images more accurately for achieving appropriate classification results with better accuracy. However, the deep learning based models have recorded satisfactory outcomes for the same.

Advancements in imaging techniques will result in enhanced classification accuracies due to better feature generalization. The most-discussed learning based techniques are considerably rooted in the preparation of a training image dataset hitherto testing the image dataset for COVID detection in order to calculate the result with vibrant accuracy also focused to reduce the processing time efficiently. Likewise, it will create a huge generality for exploration of more research in this domain in order to increase the classification performance and find a detailed description about corona virus infection levels by analysis of extracted features from CT and X-ray based methods.

Since, the corona virus is an infectious disease being dispersed by coming in contact with infected people, it also creates a consciousness of maintaining social distancing, whereas the automated deep learning based monitoring system also provides a better way by performing a screening process through advance learning based techniques.

Here, a comparison table (Table 5.1) describes with critical information about the discussed machine learning based medical imaging models.

The details in Table 5.1 show the performances of the machine learning techniques used for corona virus detection using radiological imaging techniques. Thus, the reviewed deep learning techniques are critically explored with different aspects for automated X-ray and CT scan radiological

TABLE 5.1

Comparison Table for Machine Learning Models Stand for COVID-19 Diagnosis using Radiological Imaging Techniques

Technique / Model Name	Description	Dataset Used	Radiological Imaging Type	Consequences
COVID-Net	A machine learning model used for predicting COVID-19 cases.	COVIDx	Chest X-ray	Achieved 98.9% performance accuracy for detection of corona virus disease.
CAAD	It is a Machine learning model based on ResNet architecture mainly used for Classification of COVID19 disease & anomaly detection	X-VIRAL dataset as a regular chest X-ray images & X-COVID dataset which is a COVID infected chest X-ray images	Chest X-ray	Have achieved 83.61 % performance accuracy
DeCovNet	A supervised machine learning model constructed to detect COVID infection by performing lung segmentation with 3D CNN and UNet++	499 images from CT scanning for training & 131 CT images for testing cases.	CT scan	Recorded 90.1% classification accuracy with 1.93 second for processing of single CT image
UNet++	A segmentation model rooted with deep learning methods by screening of infected cases	49096 CT images have come from 51 patients who have COVID infected & 55 patients who have some other kind of infection	CT scan	The model has achieved 98.85% performance accuracy.
ResNet50 &UNet ++	A deep learning framework for COVID detection.	CT images have been used for training the system.	CT scan	A screening System evolved for COVID detection.
COVID-ResNet	A deep learning based model using pre trained CNN with ResNet50 for COVID diagnosis.	-	X-ray	96.23 % of classification accuracy
DeTraC	A deep learning model designed with three strategies of Decomposition, transferring & Composition.	-	Chest X-ray	95.12% of classification performance

(continued)

TABLE 5.1 (Continued)

Comparison Table for Machine Learning Models Stand for COVID-19 Diagnosis using Radiological Imaging Techniques

Technique / Model Name	Description	Dataset Used	Radiological Imaging Type	Consequences
Comparison of Three Deep learning architecture Model	A deep learning model using three different architectures for COVID detection namely ResNet50, InceptionV3 & Inception-ResNetV2 for COVID detection.	-	Chest X-ray	ResNet50 with highest accuracy of 98% whereas InceptionV3 with 97% and Inception-ResNetV2 with 87%
COVIDx-Net	A deep learning system for COVID diagnosis with 7 different CNN based models such as VGG19, InceptionV3, MobileNetV2, DensNet201, ResNetV2, Inception-ResNetV2, & Xception.	50 X-ray images from 25 Corona virus infected patient cases.	X-ray	The results recorded highest performance with DensNet201 and VGG19 with 90% precision. Whereas lowest performance of 50% with Inception V3 model.

imaging detection and diagnosis methods, mainly trying to contribute to the fight against COVID-19.

5.5 Conclusion

For diagnosing corona virus infection, the X-ray and computer tomography (CT) scanning are primarily using radiology based technologies. However, restricting spread of the corona virus among the medical practitioners who regularly come in contact with infected patients is very crucial. Artificial Intelligence based machine learning techniques can play a vital role in monitoring, using a contact-less automated system for diagnosis of corona virus disease. The minimized contact between the medical team and infected person reduces the risk of infection which, in turn, is helpful to minimize the spread of corona virus.

This chapter is helpful for dealing with COVID cases along with many diversified automated learning based techniques for COVID-19 detection and diagnosis as well as for other similar infectious diseases in future. Since the computer aided detection and diagnosis of corona virus disease is mostly dependent on the classification and monitoring process, the performance outcome can be increased by enhancing the quality and quantity of training-image data for identification of COVID cases along with reduced convergence time.

References

1. Rao, A. S. S., &Vazquez, J. A. (2020). Identification of COVID-19 can be quicker through artificial intelligence framework using a mobile phone–based survey when cities and towns are under quarantine. *Infection Control & Hospital Epidemiology, 41*(7), 826–830.
2. Chung, M., Bernheim, A., Mei, X., et al. (2020). CT imaging features of 2019 novel coronavirus (2019-nCoV). *Radiology, 295*(1), 202–207.
3. Pan, L., Mu, M., Yang, P., et al. (2020). Clinical characteristics of COVID-19 patients with digestive symptoms in Hubei, China: a descriptive, cross-sectional, multicenter study. *The American Journal of Gastroenterology, 115.*
4. Nguyen, T. T. (2020). Artificial intelligence in the battle against coronavirus (COVID-19): a survey and future research directions. *Preprint, DOI, 10.*
5. Shi, F., Wang, J., Shi, J., et al. (2020). Review of artificial intelligence techniques in imaging data acquisition, segmentation and diagnosis for Covid-19. *IEEE Reviews in Biomedical Engineering.*
6. Ting, D. S. W., Carin, L., Dzau, V. et al. (2020). Digital technology and COVID-19. *Nature Medicine, 26*(4), 459–461.
7. Naudé, Wim (2020). Artificial Intelligence against COVID-19: An early review. IZA Discussion Papers, No. 13110, Institute of Labor Economics (IZA), Bonn, 8. Ai, T., Yang, Z., Hou, H., et al. (2020). Correlation of chest CT and RT-PCR testing in coronavirus disease 2019 (COVID-19) in China: A report of 1014 cases. *Radiology*, 200642.
8. Toussie, D., Voutsinas, N., Finkelstein, M., Cedillo, M. A., Manna, S., Maron, S. Z., ... & Concepcion, J. (2020). Clinical and chest radiography features determine patient outcomes in young and middle age adults with COVID-19. *Radiology*, 201754.
9. Chen, R. C. (2019). Automatic license plate recognition via sliding-window darknet-YOLO deep learning. *Image and Vision Computing, 87*, 47–56.
10. Bullock, J., Pham, K. H., Lam, C. S. N. et al. (2020). Mapping the landscape of artificial intelligence applications against COVID-19. *arXiv preprint arXiv:2003.11336.*
11. Javaid, M., Haleem, A., Vaishya, R., Bahl, S., Suman, R., & Vaish, A. (2020). Industry 4.0 technologies and their applications in fighting COVID-19 pandemic. *Diabetes & Metabolic Syndrome: Clinical Research & Reviews*, 14(4), 419–422.
12. Vaishya, R., Javaid, M., Khan, I. H., & Haleem, A. (2020). Artificial Intelligence (AI) applications for COVID-19 pandemic. *Diabetes & Metabolic Syndrome: Clinical Research & Reviews*, 14(4), 337–339.

13. Sethy, P. K., & Behera, S. K. (2020). Detection of coronavirus disease (Covid-19) based on deep features. *Preprints, 2020030300*, 2020.
14. Rahimzadeh, M., & Attar, A. (2020). A new modified deep convolutional neural network for detecting COVID-19 from x-ray images. *arXiv preprint arXiv:2004.08052*.
15. Majeed, T., Rashid, R., Ali, D., & Asaad, A. (2020). Covid-19 detection using CNN transfer learning from X-ray Images. *medRxiv*. https://doi.org/10.1101/2020.05.12.20098954.
16. Yavuz, Ü. N. A. L., & Dudak, M. N. Classification of Covid-19 dataset with some machine learning methods. *Journal of Amasya University the Institute of Sciences and Technology*, *1*(1), 30–37.
17. Wang, L., & Wong, A. (2020). COVID-Net: A tailored deep convolutional neural network design for detection of COVID-19 cases from chest -ray images. *arXiv preprintarXiv: 2003.09871*.
18. Zhang, J., Xie, Y., Li, Y., et al. (2020). Covid-19 screening on chest x-ray images using deep learning based anomaly detection. *arXiv preprint arXiv:2003.12338*.
19. Zheng, C., Deng, X., Fu, Q., et al. (2020). Deep learning-based detection for COVID-19 from chest CT using weak label. *medRxiv*. https://doi.org/10.1101/2020.05.12.20098954.
20. Chen, J., Wu, L., Zhang, J., et al. (2020). Deep learning-based model for detecting 2019 novel coronavirus pneumonia on high-resolution computed tomography: A prospective study. *MedRxiv*. https://doi.org/10.1038/s41598-020-76282-0.
21. Jin, S., Wang, B., Xu, H., et al. (2020). AI-assisted CT imaging analysis for COVID-19 screening: Building and deploying a medical AI system in four weeks. *medRxiv*. https://doi.org/10.1101/2020.03.19.20039354.
22. Farooq, M., & Hafeez, A. (2020). Covid-resnet: A deep learning framework for screening of covid19 from radiographs. *arXiv preprint arXiv:2003.14395*.
23. Abbas, A., Abdelsamea, M. M., & Gaber, M. M. (2020). Classification of COVID-19 in chest X-ray images using DeTraC deep convolutional neural network. *arXiv preprint arXiv:2003.13815*.
24. Narin, A., Kaya, C., & Pamuk, Z. (2020). Automatic detection of coronavirus disease (covid-19) using -ray images and deep convolutional neural networks. *arXiv preprint arXiv:2003.10849*.
25. Ghoshal, B., & Tucker, A. (2020). Estimating uncertainty and interpretability in deep learning for coronavirus (COVID-19) detection. *arXiv preprint arXiv:2003.10769*.
26. El-Din Hemdan, E., Shouman, M. A., & Karar, M. E. (2020). COVIDX-Net: A framework of deep learning classifiers to diagnose COVID-19 in x-ray images. *arXiv*, arXiv-2003.

6

Cardiac Health Assessment Using ANN in Diabetic Population

Manjusha Joshi, K. D. Desai, M. S. Menon, and Harish Verlekar

CONTENTS

6.1 Introduction

According to WHO reports, myocardial ischemia/infarction tops the list of causes of death over the entire globe. In the year 2015, the total number of deaths due myocardial ischemia/infarction were 15 million, and death due to diabetes was 1.6 million [1]. Episodes of myocardial ischemia/infarction are more predominant in diabetic disorder [2–10]. Diabetes was referred to as a global epidemic [2]. In type-2 diabetic disorder, the body cells are resistant to glucose and hence are unable to extract nutrients from glucose in the blood, and the energy requirement of the cells is fulfilled by the fats and proteins [3–6]. In type-2 diabetic disorder, metabolism that in normal cases uses glucose as energy currency starts using proteins and fats to acquire energy. This results in accumulation of suspended fat and calcium particles into the blood vessels, thereby reducing the lumens of blood vessels in prolonged prevalence of diabetic pathology [3–6]. This results in globally reduced blood supply due to occluded blood vessels. If the blood vessels supplying blood to the myocardium are occluded, it reduces the blood supply to the myocardium, causing myocardial ischemia that further advances to myocardial infarction (referred to as a heart attack in layman's language) [2–10].

Myocardial ischemia is the beginning of cardiac deterioration and is a reversible process, whereas myocardial infarction is final stage of deterioration and is not reversible [3–5]. Prolonged diabetic disorder causes a multitude of complications. Increased glucose levels in the blood for a long duration lead to kidney dysfunction [3–5]. To avoid this, tight glycemic control is recommended [3–5]. The diabetic subject hence maintains low blood sugar levels by restricting sugar intake. This increases the possibility of hypoglycemia. Frequent hypoglycemic episodes lead to deterioration in cardiac performance [4, 5, 9]. The ventricular depolarization and repolarization rate result in rhythmic expansion and relaxation of ventricles required for effective blood supply. Sympathetic and parasympathetic hormones control the heart relaxation and contraction intervals [7–9]. Diabetes skews the hormonal balance that reduces the ventricular depolarization interval and also makes the myocardial muscles flaccid [7–13]. Flaccidity of the myocardium culminates in reduced elasticity of the ventricular muscles and heart is unable to pump blood [7–9, 14, 17]. All the above-mentioned changes are gradual and vary in extent from person to person. There is no deterministic pattern of the complications, and the pattern and extent are highly subjective [3, 18–20].

In diabetic subjects, deterioration in cardiac performance is gradual, reversible at an early stage but not visible in clinical symptoms [2–5, 8, 9]. Hence a cardiac health assessment check at regular intervals is necessary [2–5]. The advantages of HRV analysis are many. It can assess cardiac performance before the symptoms appear and is a safe and noninvasive tool. [2–5, 14]. HRV analysis costs less than echocardiograms and takes only three to five minutes. An HRV test can be conducted by supporting paramedical staff. This saves the precious time of the cardiologists. [3] A proposed study attempts to validate the HRV indices with the currently practiced echocardiogram diagnostic index. Left Ventricular Ejection Fraction (LVEF) is the echocardiogram index that stated the mechanical performance of the left ventricle [18–21]. If the left ventricle is affected by prolonged diabetic pathology due to increased parasympathetic power, its muscles are more likely to lose their elasticity. If there is some occlusion in the blood vessels that supply blood to the left ventricle, myocardium of the left ventricle is more likely to have ischemia/infarction. In both the cases, the LVEF is reduced. Echocardiogram is a noninvasive diagnostic test that is approved by cardiologists. Compared to the HRV indices, an echocardiogram suffers from the severe limitation that it does not have preclinical assessment capability. HRV analysis can predict cardiac deterioration based on the HRV indices such as HR, SDNN, HF Power, orthostatic stress index and so forth. [2, 4, 5]. It is necessary to classify the diabetic and non-diabetic subjects based on their HRV indices. A proposed study implements the Artificial Neural Network classifier and further forms the clusters within the diabetic cohort based upon the values of the HRV indices used as feature set. Clusters are formed on the basis of deviation of HRV indices from the normal values and hence indicating the extent of cardiac function deterioration [22–24].

This chapter is arranged into sections:

Section 6.2 discusses the literature survey that shaped this study. Section 6.3 discusses the need for early diagnosis, and discusses the experiment and the requirement to conduct the experiment. Section 6.4 overviews HRV analysis. Section 6.5 states data acquisition protocol, inclusion and exclusion criterion. Section 6.6 justifies the need of classifier design and implementation. Section 6.7 states and justifies the feature set design. Section 6.8 explains the classifier design using ANN. Section 6.9 discusses cluster analysis design and implementation. Section 6.10 discusses the results of the study and its significance, and Section 6.11 discusses scope and limitation of the work.

6.2 Relevance of Early Diagnosis of Myocardial Ischemia

Myocardial ischemia/ infarction is caused by the slow death of the myocardium due to prolonged lack of nutrients. Initially the muscle will suffer from ischemia, that is, reduced blood supply. Myocardium is devoid of nutrients due to reduced blood supply and slows down the contraction and relaxation function. This condition is called hypokinetia of grade-I/II. In this stage, the slowdown in the wall velocity is visible in an echo-cardiogram. Cardiologists prescribe echo-cardiograms when the subject complains of breathlessness or fatigue. Breathlessness and fatigue are the manifestations of reduced cardiac performance at an advanced stage. Initially, as there is no symptom, there is no way to diagnose hypokinetia. This condition culminates in loss of elasticity of the heart wall.

If left ventricular myocardium suffers from prolonged grade-I/II hypokinetia, it culminates in reduced LVEF and grade-III/IV hypokinetia. Prolonged grade-III/IV hypokinetia leads to papillary muscle dysfunction culminating complications such as:

1. Reduced LVEF;
2. Chamber remodeling;
3. Volumetric changes in heart chambers;
4. Aneurysm, and
5. Severe dilation.

The myocardium can be recovered at the ischemic stage if diagnosed, and blood supply can be improved by treatment or intervention as deemed fit by the cardiologist. Alternatively, loss of movement of myocardium is compensated by the nearby muscles that make a condition called dyskinesia, where the movement of the ventricle goes off-centric and fails to function in normal fashion, leading to the same results and listed above.

This discussion clearly explains the need of early diagnostic practices. By periodic acquisition of HRV reports in prevailing diabetic conditions, the mortality rate and morbidity can be controlled, thereby improving the quality of life of a diabetic subject.

6.3 Materials and Methods

Every subject is briefly informed about the study before acquiring the data. As the data acquisition is non-invasive, written permission from the subject is not mandatory, according to the Helsinki WMA declaration. ECG data samples of 3–5 minutes duration are acquired from diabetic and non-diabetic and non-hypertensive cohorts for the HRV analysis. If ECG samples are acquired for three minutes, at least 128 R-R samples of II Lead ECG can be availed for HRV analysis [2]. ECG samples of subjects are acquired by ensuring the subject is at rest and is relaxing mentally by prior instruction. This is possible by acquiring the sample by keeping the patient in a supine position as per the protocol of data acquisition for HRV analysis. HRV analysis of control group and diabetic subjects is computed. The ECG signal is acquired using LABVIEW. The acquired ECG signal includes 50 Hz supply interference and high frequency cardiac muscle artefact. elimination of noise from the signal to weed out DC interference (low frequency signal) and muscle artefact (high frequency signal) using MATLAB program at the back end. ECG samples care processed to acquire R-R interval samples. These samples are used to compute different HRV indices.

6.3.1 HRV Analysis Tool

The HRV simulator by PHYSIONET is used for analysis [2, 4 and 5]. Figure 6.1 shows the result sheet. The simulator provides the indices in the time and frequency domain as well as the nonlinear indices. The features used for classification in the chapter uses three indices as heart rate, SDNN (i.e., the heart rate variability) and parasympathetic power. These indices of diabetic and normal subjects are the feature set of the classifier [2, 4 and 5].

6.4 Overview of HRV Analysis

A healthy heart responds to physiological, physical and psychological changes in the body, and the basal heart rate (HR) is modified as required by the body. Impaired hearts cannot cope with the varying demands of blood supply by different activities of body. The impaired heart is not able to supply more blood when the body demands it. This leads to reduced blood supply to the entire body. As a defense mechanism, diabetic subjects are observed to have higher basal heart rates and the condition is referred as basal tachycardia [2]. Increase in heart rate marks the onset of cardiac deterioration in diabetic subjects. This feature is one of the prominent distinguishing features of HRV analysis in diabetic pathology.

The inability of the heart to change the heart rate as per the body demands results in reduced variability in heart rate. This is called as SDNN, that is, the standard deviation of N-N interval. N refers to the start point of the PQRS curve. Since it is easy to detect R in automatic detection, we refer to this as variation in R-R interval. The SDNN value is very high in a healthy heart, and the value progressively goes lower. With prevailing diabetes, the SDNN value is reduced [2]. Reduced SDNN is also positively correlated by computing the orthostatic stress index. This parameter is quantitative evaluation of adaptability of the heart to changing demands of the blood supply [2].

The HRV analysis derives diagnostic indices from the spectral analysis of R-R intervals. Fourier analysis of the acquired R-R intervals is computed to evaluate the power spectral density of the three frequency bands of interest. Autoregressive analysis gives information about three frequency bands such as the VLF band, 0.0–0.04Hz, LF band, 0.04–0.15Hz and HF band, 0.15 to 0.4Hz [5]. HF band power indicates the parasympathetic power, and LF band power indicates the sympathetic power generated by the central autonomous system. Heart rate is controlled by complex interplay of the two powers. These powers have dominance depending upon the hormonal stimulus from the autonomous nervous system. The cardiac response results from the autonomous nervous system, and autonomous nervous response cannot be modulated by any pharmaceutical intervention. This feature of HRV analysis is unique and powerful. No other diagnostic method can evaluate the extent of skewness that tampers the autonomous neural balance. HRV analysis can state whether there is dominance of parasympathetic power in a diabetic subject. The HRV simulator analyses the power distribution in different frequency bands using Fourier analysis and can enumerate the power of the two frequency bands that are associated with sympathetic and parasympathetic hormonal inputs at preganglionic stage. This enumeration can state the extent of skewness of the hormonal imbalance, and therefore HRV analysis has the diagnostic ability to assess cardiac function deterioration at the preclinical level. [2–5, 15]

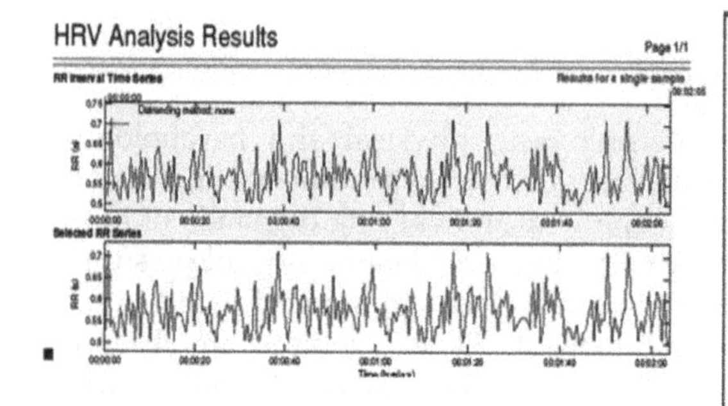

Variable	Units	Value
Mean RR*	(ms)	568.4
STD RR (SDNN)	(ms)	48.7
Mean HR*	(1/min)	106.30
STD HR	(1/min)	8.68
RMSSD	(ms)	69.6
NN50	(count)	107
pNN50	(%)	49.1
RR triangular index		11.526
TINN	(ms)	220.0

FIGURE 6.1A
Tachogram from HRV Report.

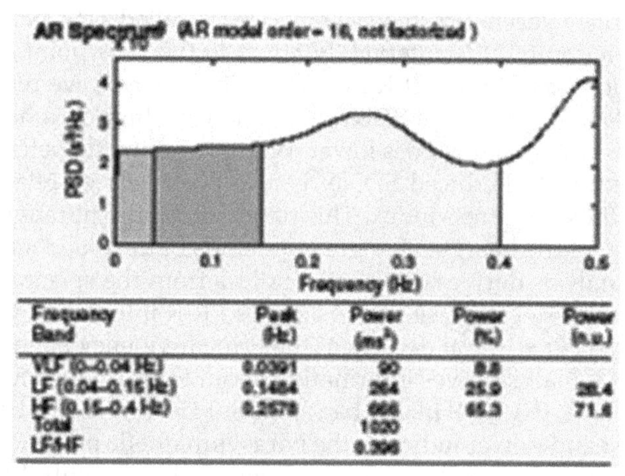

Frequency Band	Peak (Hz)	Power (ms²)	Power (%)	Power (n.u.)
VLF (0–0.04 Hz)	0.0391	90	8.8	
LF (0.04–0.15 Hz)	0.1484	264	25.9	28.4
HF (0.15–0.4 Hz)	0.2578	666	65.3	71.6
Total		1020		
LF/HF		0.396		

FIGURE 6.1B
HRV Indices from AR Analysis of R-R Intervals.

The simulation results of a sample HRV analysis are shown in the Figure 6.1A. A tachogram of the variation in R-R interval variations is shown in Figure 6.1A. Figure 6.1B shows the AR analysis of R-R intervals that are considered in the study.

6.5 Data Acquisition Protocol, Inclusion and Exclusion Criterion

Study is carried out on diabetic and non-hypertensive subjects as disease cohort and non-diabetic and non-hypertensive subjects as a control cohort that visit the hospital for checkups or were admitted to the hospital. The II LEAD ECG and echo-cardiogram are acquired on the same day. Data from a 27-member control group and 47-member diabetic group are recorded. [23]

1. All the cases were recorded from Fortis-S L Raheja Hospital.
2. To ensure maximum variation in data samples, subjects are chosen as they register and not filtered by any medical staff. The records are collected in the morning from 10 a.m. to 2 p.m.
3. All the subjects are above 25 years of age.
4. The ECG acquisition equipment is same.
5. The control group consists of non-diabetic and non-hypertensive subjects.
6. The diabetic subjects have at least 5 years of prevailing diabetes.
7. The clinical glycemic control record is not mandatory in diabetic cases.
8. Both male female cases are included.

The exclusion criterion states:

1. Subjects who are younger than 25 years age.
2. Subjects suffering from type-1 diabetes.
3. Subjects with less than 5 years of diabetes history in study group.
4. Subjects with known history of electrolyte imbalance related ECG abnormalities.
5. Subjects with known history of Digitalis induced ECG abnormalities.
6. Subjects that are only diabetic and with no other complications are considered.

A clarification about Digitalis is necessary. It is a medicine that regulates the heartbeat and is used to treat certain types of arrhythmia. Exclusion of cases that are on Digitalis medication is necessary as the autonomous rhythm is no more observable if the subject is under this medication.

6.6 Need of Classifier

The central autonomous system fires the pacemaker or the SA node that triggers the pulse resulting in an R peak. The activation for the trigger is initiated by any of the eight different inputs listed below [2 and 10].

1. Baroreceptors located in the peripheral organs indicate reduced Arterial Blood Pressure (ABP).

2. Volume receptors located in the alveoli of lungs indicate reduced instantaneous lung volume (ILV).
3. The chemoreceptors located in the central nervous system indicate variation in hormonal level from parasympathetic and sympathetic stimulations indicating that blood is necessary when sympathetic stimulation exceeds parasympathetic stimulation.
4. Reduced oxygen concentration level in the blood plasma from the chemoreceptors located in the peripheral circulatory system.
5. Temperature changes from the thermo-sensors located all over the body.
6. Increased stress hormonal level from the chemoreceptor located in the brain.
7. The relaxation status of the stretch receptors located in the heart wall to check when ventricular diastole has occurred before.
8. The time at which the previous R peak fires.

When the input trigger has more power than the qualifying threshold level, SA node triggers R peak. Clearly, the system is quite complex with eight closed loop controls. Simplification of the system to study only the hormonal variation is necessary. If the subject is resting in a calm cool place and is instructed to relax, it can be safely assumed that:

1. Blood pressure of the subject is controlled.
2. Lung volume does not vary due to regular breathing in resting position.
3. Since subject is resting, oxygen level in the blood is constant.
4. Cool controlled temperature in the room controls the temperature variations.
5. Subject is instructed to relax so the mental stress hormones are not triggered.
6. Due to resting position, stretch receptors on the heart wall are responding in tandem with the ventricular contraction and relaxation interval.
7. The Last R peak interval due to resting position is controlled.

So we can conclude that autonomous firing of SA node of heart is continuously controlled by sympathetic and parasympathetic hormonal secretion in the given circumstances. While the subject is resting, parasympathetic power dominates. In diabetic subjects, the parasympathetic power dominates. In different stages of diabetes, the extent of domination varies, and the exact proportion of the hormonal imbalance does not follow any fixed pattern and is highly subjective. Hence the R-R interval variation, and hence the HRV analysis indices, cannot be modelled by deterministic process. Classifier attempts to identify how the feature set of diabetic subjects is different. In other words, this problem is a system identification of cardiac function of diabetic subjects. For indeterministic system equation, artificial Neural Network (ANN) is an effective tool.

6.7 Feature Set Design

As already stated, there is no fixed course of changes in the diabetic pathology that can deterministically state the course and extent of complications. Prolonged diabetic disorder causes different types of complications. There is no pattern of onset of complications of target organs. The prevalence and extent of degradation is completely random and subjective. Hence, it is very crucial to identify the robust feature set that can effectively classify all the subjects at different stages of diabetes. Randomness and variety of cases is ensured by the data-acquisition protocol. The data is acquired as and when the diabetic subjects have reported for consultation at the hospital.

As there is large variation in the parameter values of the subjects depending upon the extent of performance deterioration, feature set evaluation based on the values of the feature set is essential. The quantitative analysis of feature set values is equally essential to validate the feature set, and that is ensured by cluster analysis performed after classifier implementation. Cluster analysis is necessarily an unsupervised analysis. In this case since cardiac performance is marked by LVEF, the accuracy of cluster analysis is possible.

6.8 ANN Classifier Design

Machine learning tools like ANN are useful in classification of uncertain or subjective data. Accurate and adequate feature selection will result in accurate classification [21]. Feature set is identified from the domain knowledge. It is crucial to validate the features by implementing the classifier with high constraints on performance. The classifier should have high accuracy with minimum error in Type-I and Type-II. Type-I error signifies the number of the misclassified data that identifies normal parameters as risky, and Type-II is vice versa. Both types of errors (false positive and false negative) are equally risky for the subject who is misclassified. Minimum Type-I and II errors increase the sensitivity and specificity.

Basic steps of preprocessing of data required for a classifier are listed as

1. Acquiring raw dataset;
2. Preprocessing of data;

3. Feature set design;
4. ANN classifier.

The raw dataset contains the different HRV indices of normal and diabetic subjects. The candidate features are heart rate, heart rate variability (SDNN) and parasympathetic power. Interdependency between the candidate features is checked by student's t-test, and the p values are found to be less than 0.05. Hence, it is ascertained candidate parameters minimal and essential features [21] [22].

Data values are normalized and randomized for creating a random input data set. Pearson's correlation index computed for the candidate parameters to ensure that the feature space is not correlated and independent. Normal and deteriorated cardiac performances are set with values as 0 and 1 respectively for the target set. The control subjects cannot be regarded as healthy individuals. They have visited the hospital for some ailment or routine health check. So it may be possible that some of the control group outcome can be 0, leading to misclassification. Such cases are eliminated at the preprocessing level.

In a supervised classifier, the classifier outcome is considered as a desired signal. The classifier implements the perceptron learning rule. The error in current iteration modifies the synaptic weights associated with the input. To ascertain the significance of the feature set, weight vector modification based on supervised data is the most suitable configuration for implementation of a classifier [25]. Error-back propagation algorithm is used as most suitable for weight optimization due to error feedback. Figure 6.2 shows the architecture of the error-back propagation algorithm with only one neuron in the output layer for a binary classifier. Scaled conjugate grading algorithm is used for better accuracy and less memory usage. This algorithm solves many parameter systems as simultaneous linear equations with small round off errors and converges to desired values with a small number of iterations. Hence the algorithm is computationally efficient. The classifier design is based on pattern recognition since the process is considered as random. ANN is programmed for a pattern recognition tool. The reason for using pattern recognition techniques is justified because of the functioning of the heart is a complex non- stationary process with no deterministic equation, but it certainly has a specific pattern for diabetic and/or hypertensive pathology.

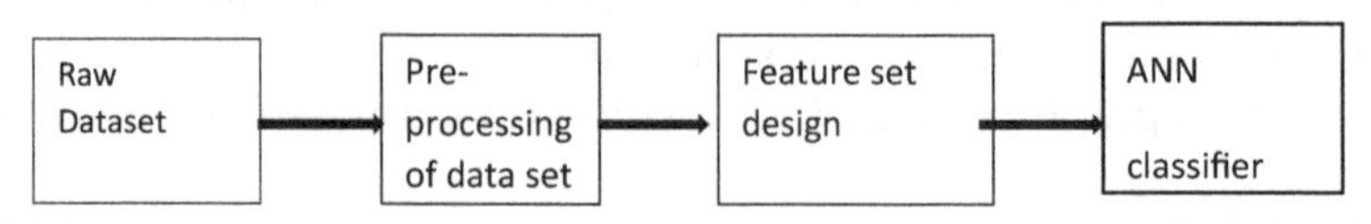

FIGURE 6.2
Error Back Propagation using ANN.

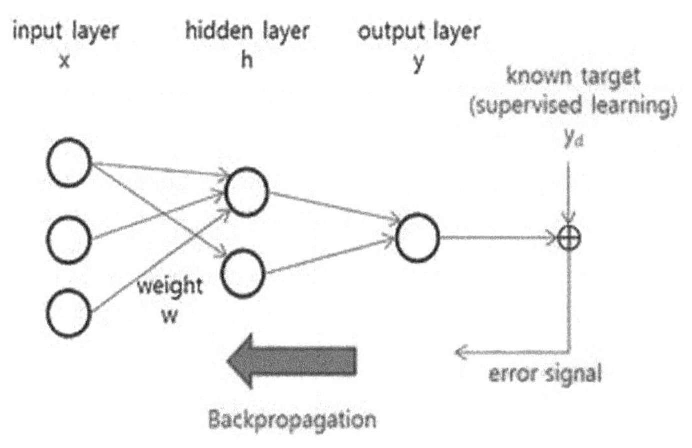

FIGURE 6.3
ANN Classifier.

Left Ventricular Ejection Fraction (LVEF) of every subject is recorded from the echo-cardiogram. Since the echo-cardiogram is an established diagnostic tool, it can be considered as an authentic outcome to validate the feature set of the HRV analysis. The LVEF is the most dependable factor as it gives the mechanical performance output of the myocardium. The value of LVEF is the manifestation of the prolonged dominance of norepinephrine that makes the heart muscles flaccid and decreases the depolarization rate. It is the suitable value of the desired signal to tune the weight vector of the classifier design. Supervised classifier design is illustrated in Figure 6.3. With a known outcome of the target set, supervised artificial neural network algorithm can be used. Supervised ANN algorithm has the greatest advantage of high performance.

The ANN classifier checks accuracy and performance by comparing with the outcome of the target data set. True positive rate (TPR) and false positive rate (FPR) and the receiver operating characteristics (ROC) for the training, test and validation data set are indicators used in this study. The confusion matrix of the classifier computed the classifier accuracy of input, test and validation data set.

6.9 Cluster Analysis

Cluster analysis is performed by k-means clustering technique. This technique partitions n number of data points into k partitions where n>k. The method is also known as nearest centroid classifier [26]. The analysis begins with a plot of different points of occurrences versus the parameter under observation. Looking at the distribution, the groups of highest incidence can be visually analyzed. A centroid point is chosen for every cluster of points. The centroid is a point that represents the cluster with zero deviation. The nearby points with smaller deviations populate the cluster. As the data points move away from the centroid, they lose the corresponding cluster identity. The threshold value of the minimum distance from the centroid depends upon the domain knowledge. In any data set, largest data points in one cluster are the strongest representative of that class. Data points that do not belong to any class may also exist, and they may be the outliers in that class. Choice of centroid is based on the maximum points populating the particular spot in the distribution graph. Too small a centroid value does not analyze the clusters and characterization of the given parameter for the sample space is not accurate. Too large a number of clusters causes over-modelling of the sample space. The elbow method uses a parameter called "within cluster sum of square" (WCSS), plotted against the number of clusters. The optimum number of clusters is indicated at the point of sharp decrease in the value on the X axis where, number of clusters are represented.

In semi-supervised cluster analysis, the validation of the clusters can be possible if the outcome of the study is known. In the proposed study, the LVEF of the subjects is available. The same values can be checked for the high-risk cluster from the sample space and hence the validation of the feature set is possible.

6.10 Results and Discussion

Table 6.1 shows the HRV indices-heart rate, heart rate variability (SDNN) and the parasympathetic power (HF Power) of the control group and the diabetic group. The average value of heart rate and HF power for the diabetic cohort is higher than the average value of the normal cohort. The SDNN of normal subjects is higher than the diabetic subjects.

The p-value indicates that the three parameters are statistically independent. Table 6.2 shows the p-value of one tailed t-test of unequal variance

TABLE 6.1

Average Heart Rate of Control Group and the Diabetic Cohort

Cohort Type	Average SDNN	Average Heart Rate	Average HF power
Normal	45.36	66.34	0.6684
Diabetic	38.36	85.66	0.5389

TABLE 6.2

T-test for Entire Data Set

Category	Heart Rate	SDNN	HF Power
p-values	0.00222	0.00812	0.04693

TABLE 6.3

Pearson's Correlation Index for Entire Data Set

Category	Heart Rate and SDNN	Heart Rate and HF Power	SDNN and HF Power
Pearson's Correlation Index	0.0022	0.044	0.00812

between normal and diabetic cohort. It can be observed that p-value is much below 0.05. The t-test results are tabulated to show the data of the indices are not dependent on each other. Table 6.3 shows the Pearson's correlation index values indicating that the changes in the data are not interrelated.

The candidate values for the subjects in the normal and diabetic cohort are observed to be highly varying. This is due to the fact that biological data is highly subjective. The values are found to be categorically different in diabetic subjects, depending to a large extent on the duration of diabetes, glycemic control and lifestyle of the diabetic subjects. The overlap in the candidate values can be seen in the Figures 6.4A, 6.4B and 6.4C shown below.

The data distribution for the candidate features is shown in the Figure 6.4A to Figure 6.4C. Samples of some 20 control subjects and disease subjects are plotted on the X-axis, and normalized HR, SDNN and HF Power are plotted on the Y-axis. There is no clear differentiation between the values of the indices for the normal and diabetic cohorts. A lot of overlap in the values of the indices can be observed. It can be concluded that the classifier does not follow any deterministic equation or clear pattern. Artificial Neural Networks are effective tools in such types of classification that can learn from the multivariate pattern [22–24]. It can be concluded after observing the trends of candidate values that the design of the classifier using ANN is justified.

The ANN classifier configuration is shown in Figure 6.5A. The candidate parameter is four (heart rate, SDNN, HF Power and LVEF), the target class is two (normal and diabetic).

Figure 6.5B represents the performance of the classifier by accuracy of the training, validation and test data. The average of all is plotted in the last block. Any row in the confusion matrix shows the false negative, false positive and true positive values respectively. The first row represents the values for class-1, that is, for a normal cohort, and the second row represents the same for class-2, that is, for disease cohort. The third row represents the average of

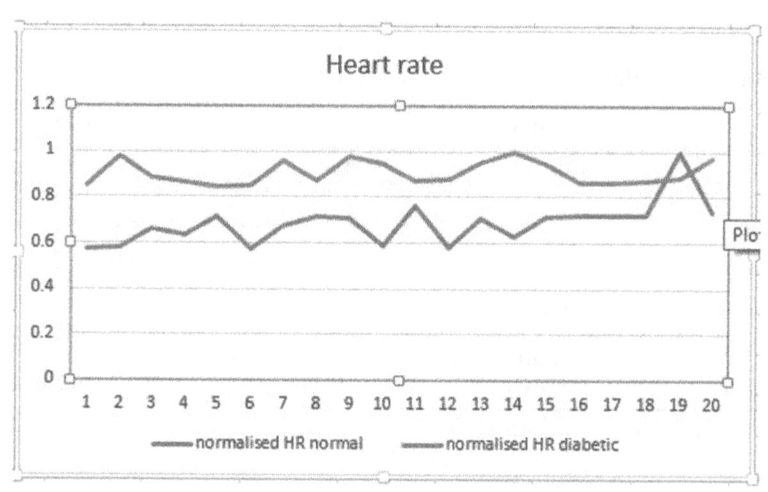

FIGURE 6.4A
Heart Rate of the Two Cohorts.

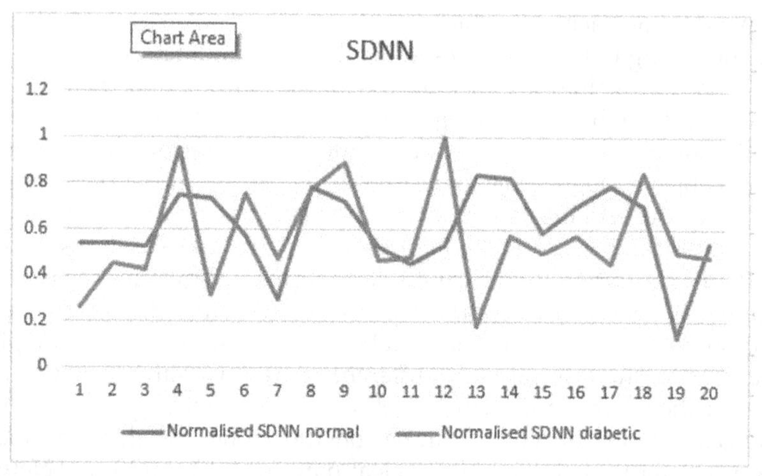

FIGURE 6.4B
Heart Rate Variability (SDNN) of the Two Cohorts.

results for both the classes. NaN value can be seen in the last row as there are zero values for false positives of both the classes. The classifier accuracy can be increased up to some extent by increasing number of neurons. Figure 6.5C represents the performance of training data, test data and validation data. Minimum error at 41st epoch is specified as 10^{-5}.

From comparing the above results, it can be seen that the ANN classifier can be used as a tool to test unknown targets and to check whether the subject is diabetic or nondiabetic.

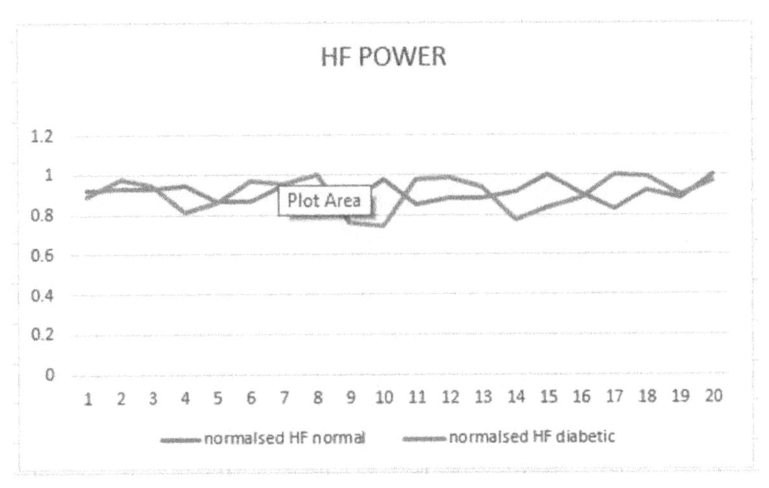

FIGURE 6.4C
HF Power of the Two Cohorts.

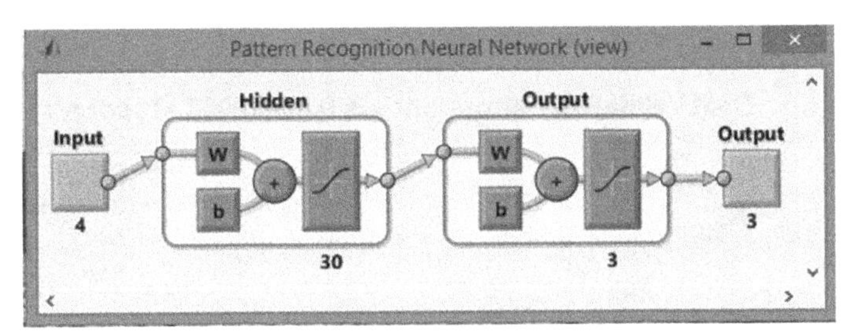

FIGURE 6.5A
Configuration of ANN.

The performance of the classifier can be regarded as very excellent as the error convergence is seen at a much lower number of epochs from Figure 6.5C. Hence, it can be concluded that the designed classifier can be a reliable tool to classify the diabetic and nondiabetic groups based on their cardiac parameters. Also, the number of neurons in the classifier need not be increased.

Further cluster analysis gives information about the trend of the data within the diabetic group. The K-NN clustering method is used. Feature set validation is one significant outcome of cluster analysis. The elbow method is used to ascertain the number of clusters for each feature. The elbow method plot and case-wise distribution of diabetic subjects versus HR, HF power and SDNN are plotted in Figure 6.6A, 6.6B and 6.6C. The left panel shows the elbow method plot for the corresponding feature cluster plot. The distribution of the features show that there are large variations of the feature set values across the diabetic cohort.

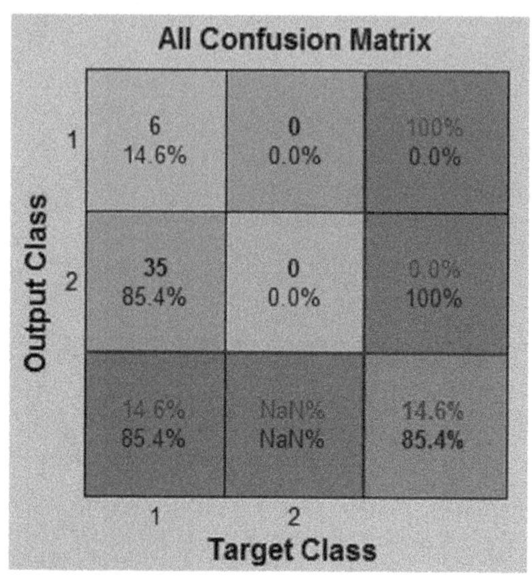

FIGURE 6.5B
Confusion Matrix of ANN Classifier.

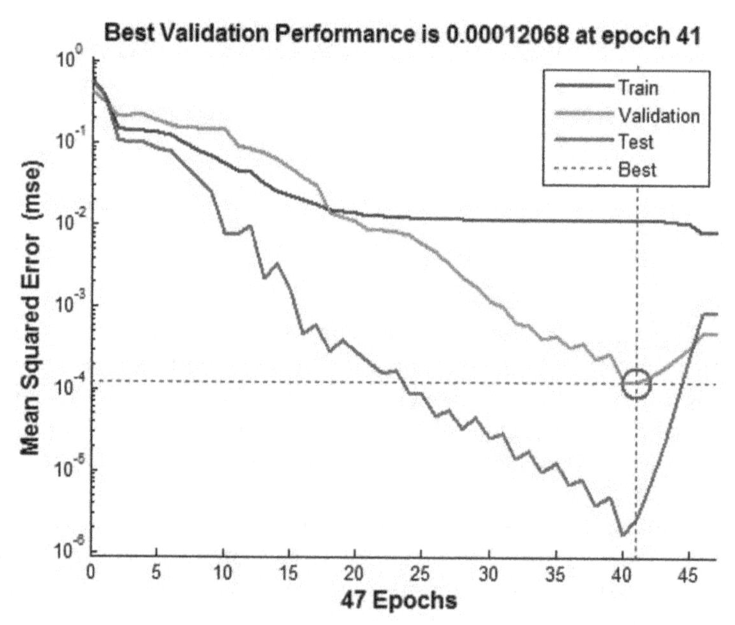

FIGURE 6.5C
Performance Graph of the Training, Validation and Testing.

Sample data for cluster-2 is tabulated in Table 6.4 to understand one of the clusters. It can be seen from Figure 6.7, that cluster-1 represents the healthiest cardiac health of the sample population, whereas cluster-2 represents the

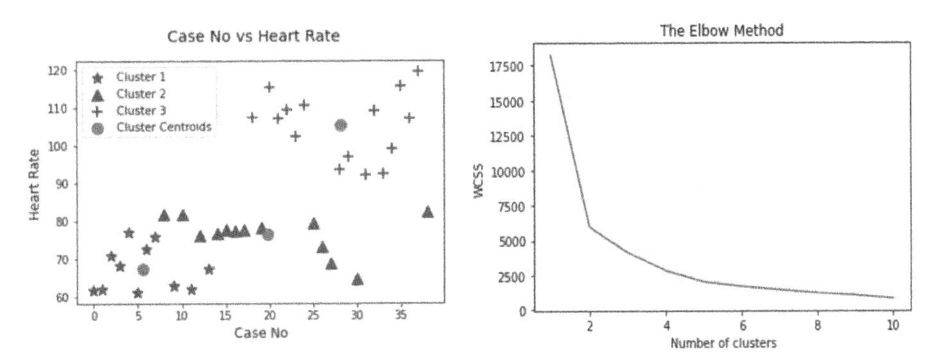

FIGURE 6.6A
Elbow Method Plot and the Cluster Distribution for HR.

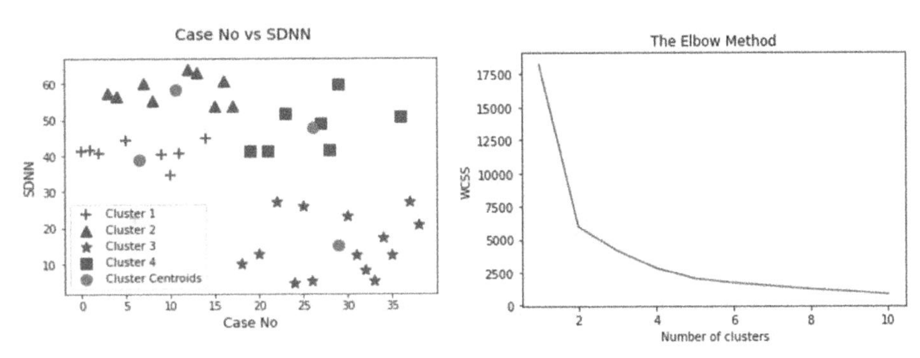

FIGURE 6.6B
Elbow Method Plot and the Cluster Distribution for SDNN.

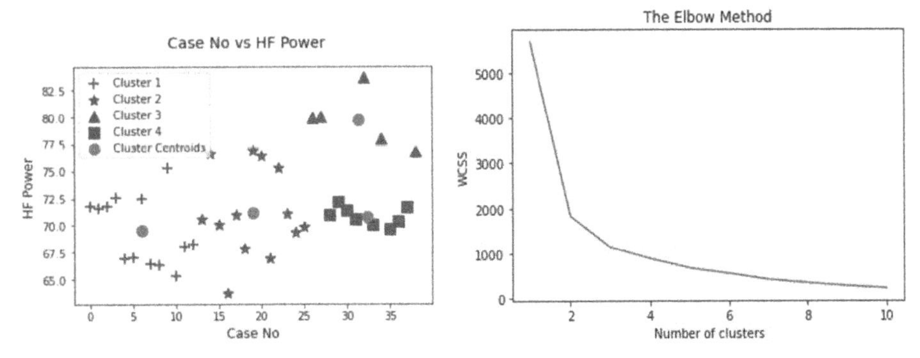

FIGURE 6.6C
Elbow Method Plot and the Cluster Distribution for HF Power.

most deteriorated cardiac health in the sample population. Clusters-3 and 4 are positioned in such a way that the parameters are quite deviated from normal values. From the plot it can be clear that cluster-2 represents HR ranging from 90 to 110, SDNN ranging from 10 to 20 and HF power ranging from 70 to 82.5. The identified range of the feature set is validated by LVEF. Table 6.4

TABLE 6.4

Features from HRV Analysis and LVEF from Echo-cardiogram for Cluster-2

Serial Number	Heart Rate	SDNN	HF Power	LVEF
1	115.36	12.7	76.4	0.32
2	110.37	4.7	69.3	0.47
3	73.14	5.3	79.9	0.19
4	92.04	12.6	70.5	0.6
5	109.17	8.3	83.6	0.25
6	92.19	5.2	70	0.56
7	99.1	17.2	78	0.41
8	115.28	12.4	69.6	0.2
9	72.42	22.7	77.4	0.56
10	107.0	10.2	67.8	0.58

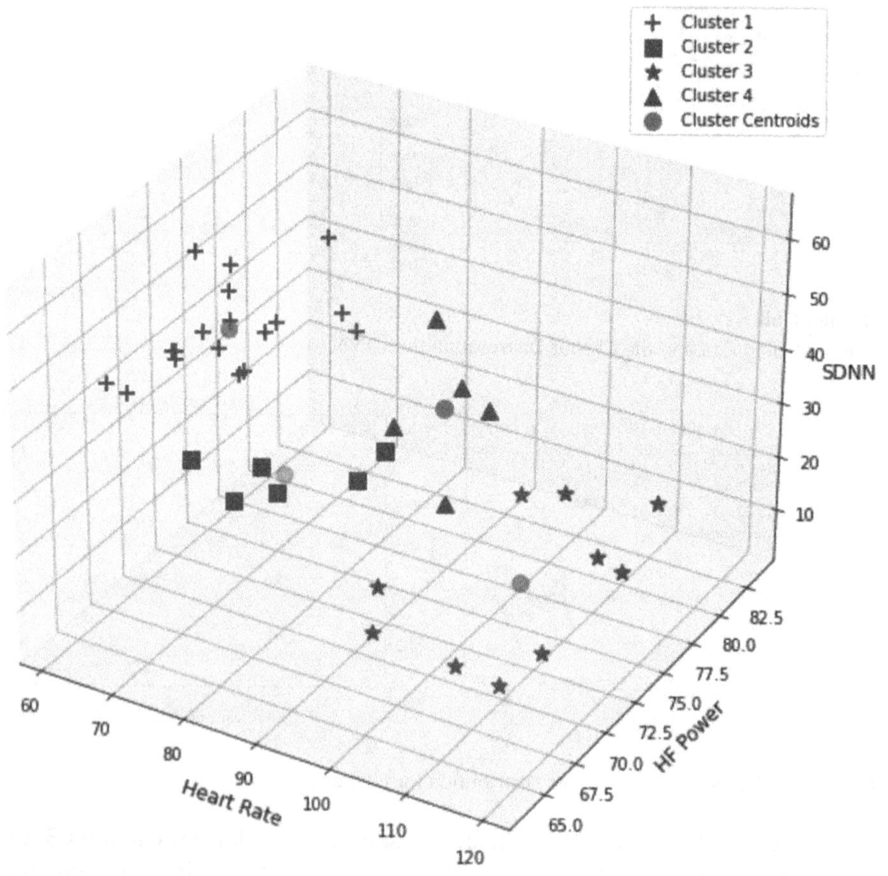

FIGURE 6.7
Cluster Plot for all the Three Parameters Together.

shows the feature set along with LVEF. Most of the cases show the LVEF value quite low, indicating that the cardiac performance has deteriorated. It can be concluded that the HRV features of cluster-2 are validated for high cardiac risk. In future, without the echocardiogram test, if the candidate feature values are in the above-mentioned range, then the subject can be considered to have potential cardiac risk.

6.11 Scope and Limitations

The authors limit the manuscript to only one method of classifier implementation and for cluster analysis. The same can be extended for different implementation methods. The authors discuss the risk stratification and validation of the feature set for only a high-risk cluster. The same can be discussed for rest of the clusters also.

References

[1] World Health Organization Statistical Information System (WHOSIS). Cardiovascular Disease Statistics. 2009. Available from www3.who.int/whosis/menu.cfm.

[2] Manjusha Joshi. "Study of myocardial ischemia implying echo-images and Heart Rate Variability data." PhD Dissertation, Chapter 1 Introduction, NMIMS deemed University, November 2015.

[3] Zi-Hui Tang, Fangfang Zeng, Zhongtao Li, & Linuo Zhou. "Association and predictive value analysis for resting heart rate and diabetes mellitus on cardiovascular autonomic neuropathy in general population." *Journal of Diabetes Research*. Vol. 2014, Article ID 215473, 7 pages. http://dx.doi.org/10.1155/2014/215473.

[4] Manjusha Joshi, K.D. Desai, & M.S. Menon. "Poincare plot used as a confirmative tool in diagnosis of LV diastolic dysfunction for diabetic and hypertensive patients." American Journal of Engineering Research, 2(9) 2013: 81–86.

[5] Manjusha Joshi, K.D. Desai, & M.S. Menon. "Correlation between heart rate variability (SDNN) and echocardiogram finding-LVEF for diabetic subjects with and without hypertension." 2015. www.britishjr.org/index.php/OJR.

[6] Arthur C. Guyton & John E. Hall, "Insulin, glucagon, and diabetes mellitus." *The Textbook of Medial Physiology, 11th edn*. (2008) India: Elsevier: 116.

[7] Emily B. Schroeder, Lloyd E. Chambless, Duanping Liao, Ronald J. Prineas, Gregory W. Evans, Wayne D. Rosamond, & Gerardo Heiss. "Diabetes, glucose, insulin, and heart rate variability – The atherosclerosis risk in communities (ARIC) study. Pathophysiology / Complications." *Pathophysiology / Complications, Diabetes Care*, 28(3), 2005.

[8] Betsy B. Dokken. "The pathophysiology of cardiovascular disease and diabetes: Beyond blood pressure and lipids." *From Research to Practise, Diabetes Spectrum*. 21(3), 2008.

[9] Marc Dweck, Ian W. Campbell, Douglas Miller, & C. Mark Francis. "Clinical Aspects of silent myocardial ischaemia: With particular reference to diabetes mellitus." *British Journal of Diabetes & Vascular Disease*, 9, 2009: 110. DOI:10.1177/1474651409105249.

[10] M. Joshi, K.D. Desai, & M.S. Menon. "Mathematical model of sino-atrial node used in assessment of neuropathy and cardiac health in diabetics." *Biomedical Engineering Research*, 4(2) 2015: 6–14.

[11] I. Antelmi, A.T. Yamada, C.N. Hsin, J.M. Tsu Tsui, C.J. Grupi, & A.J. Mansur. "Influence of parasympathetic modulation in doppler mitral inflow velocity in individuals without heart disease." NCBI-US National Library of Medicine, National Institutes of Health 2010 July 23 (7): 762–765. doi: 10.1016/j.echo.2010.04.007. Epub 2010 May 15.

[12] Alona Rudchenko, Eli Akude, & Ellis D. Cooper "Synapses on sympathetic neurons and parasympathetic neurons differ in their vulnerability to diabetes." *The Journal of Neuroscience*, 34(26) 2014: 8865–8874.

[13] F. Infusino, Pitocco, D., F. Zaccardi, G. Scavone, I. Coviello, R. Nerla, R. Mollo et al. "Low glucose blood levels are associated with abnormal cardiac sympathovagal balance in type 2 Diabetic patients with coronary artery disease." *European Review of Medical and Pharmacological Sciences*, 14(3), 2010: 203–207.

[14] Viktor Stoikov, Stevan Ilić, Marina Deljanin Ilić, Aleksandar Nikolić, & Vojislava Mitić. "Impact of diabetes on heart rate variability and left ventricular function in patients after Myocardial Infarction." Institute for Prevention, Treatment and Rehabilitation of Rheumatic and Cardiovascular Diseases. *Medicine and Biology*, 12(3), 2005: 130–134.

[15] Konstantinos D. Rizas, Tuomo Nieminen, Petra Barthel, Christine S. Zürn, Mika Kähönen, Jari Viik, Terho Lehtimäki, Kjell Nikus, Christian Eick, Tim O. Greiner, Hans P. Wendel, Peter Seizer, Jürgen Schreieck, Meinrad Gawaz, Georg Schmidt, & Axel Bauer. "Sympathetic activity–associated periodic repolarization dynamics predict mortality following myocardial infarction." *Journal of Clinical Investigation*, 124(4), 2014: 1770–1780.

[16] Farns J. Th. Wackers, Lawrence H. Young, Silvio E. Inzuchchi, et al. "Detection of silent myocardial ischemia in asymptotic diabetic subjects. The DIAD study." *Diabetic Care*, January 2005.

[17] Tushar Anil Parlikar. "Modeling and monitoring of cardiovascular dynamics for patients in critical care." Ph.D. Dissertation, Department of Electrical Engineering and Computer Science, Massachusetts Institute of Technology. June 2007.

[18] Paul Coulon, Antoine Cremer, Georgios Papaioannou & Emilie Jan, "ECG detection of left ventricular hypertrophy: the simpler, the better?" *Journal of Hypertan tsion*,30(5), 2012 May: 990–996. doi: 10.1097/HJH.0b013e3283524961.

[19] Gerard J. King, Jerome B. Foley, Faisal Almane, Peter A. Crean & Michael J. Walsh. "Early diastolic filling dynamics in diastolic dysfunction." *Cardiovascular Ultrasound*. www.cardiovascularultrasound.com/content/1/1/9.

[20] Erbel, R., Schweizer, P. Krebs, W., Langen, H.J., Meyer, J., & Effert, S. "Effects of heart rate changes on left ventricular volume and ejection fraction: A

2-dimensional echocardiographic study." *The Journal of Clinical Investigation.* 53(4), February 1984: 590–597.

[21] J.S. Smith, M.K. Cahalan, D.J. Benefiel, B.F. Byrd, F.W. Lurz, W.A. Shapiro, M.F. Roizen, A. Bouchard & N.B. Schiller. "Intraoperative detection of myocardial ischemia in high-risk patients: electrocardiography versus two-dimensional transesophageal echocardiography." *American Heart Journal.* https://circ.ahajournals.org/content/72/5/1015.short.

[22] Isabelle Guyon & André Elisseeff, "An introduction to variable and feature selection." *Journal of Machine Learning Research* 3, 2003: 1157–1182.

[23] Thierry Denoeux, "A neural network classifier based on Dempster-Shafer Theory." *IEEE Transactions on Systems, Man, and Cybernetics – Part A: Systems and Humans,* 30(2), March 2000: 131–150.

[24] B. Yegnanarayana. "Artificial neural networks for pattern recognition." *Scidhanci,* Vol. 19, Part 2, April 1994: 189–238.

[25] Rama Kishore & Taranjit Kaur. "Backpropagation algorithm: An artificial neural network approach for pattern recognition." *International Journal of Scientific & Engineering Research,* 3(6), June 2012. 1 ISSN 2229-5518.

[26] Tapas Kanungo, David M. Mount, Nathan S. Netanyahu, Christine D. Piatko, Ruth Silverman, & Angela Y. Wu. "An efficient k-means clustering algorithm: Analysis and implementation." *IEEE Transactions on Pattern Analysis and Machine Intelligence,* 24(7), 2002.

7

Efficient, Accurate and Early Detection of Myocardial Infarction Using Machine Learning

Nusrat Parveen and Satish R. Devane

CONTENTS

7.1 Introduction

The advancement of technical power represented by Moore's Law offers the potential for sanctioning less expensive medical devices and systems. There are arguments that positive technology impacts in medication occur most promptly once innovators augment the abilities of, and collaborate with, caregivers instead of seeking to displace them. In short, a technological "push" can continue within the difficult stylish application space, however, disruption can occur through wider application of lower-cost technologies forced by the user [1].

In the healthcare trade, usually diagnostic analysis culminates with the approval of health practitioners' scientific and technical knowledge and practice. Computer-aided design performs a primary role inside clinical discipline. Amongst all harmful sicknesses, coronary heart attacks are taken into consideration as the most widespread. Health-care workers study Myocardial Infarction (MI), and the accumulated records of heart patients, their ailment development and manifestation, but workers are increasingly describing sufferers with commonplace affliction who have normal signs and indications.

Scientific information is still fact-rich but information-poor. Consequently, diagnosing an affected person efficiently with the idea of time being a necessity, time is necessary for clinical assistance. A wrong diagnosis done with the aid of doctors can become fatal for the affected person. The best and correct diagnosis of coronary heart disorder is the dominant biomedical trouble.

Every year heart ailments cause tens of millions of deaths globally. Many techniques and tools have been developed for coronary heart disease predictions by medical doctors. Researchers have made efforts to expand the automated diagnosis systems in order that accurate diagnosis ought to take place. Among these, the automated machine, the usage of data mining and an AI-based total approach is the recent one used in automated prognosis.

Contemporary investigation and techniques are insufficient for correct diagnosis of myocardial infarction (MI). In addition, as for beginning doctors, their experience isn't sufficient for proper prognosis of MI. The prevailing researches have invented many machines that gain knowledge totally based on the approaches of novice doctors to assist diagnosis, but the time required and the correctness of those methods depend on the parameters given to the machine. As a result, the principal drawback of research to date about the machine acquiring information for diagnosis is the software of the classification technique for MI prediction. The motivation of the research is to develop a potent computer-aided intelligent prognosis by the use of ML techniques to be able to aid doctors in making accurate decisions regarding prognosis. In addition, the usage of patients' history statistics by those who had MI and the availability of newly invented wearable gadgets, are imparting the actual-time health parameters of someone in order to assist with a prognosis of early possibility of having MI.

7.1.1 Myocardial Infarction

The coronary movement is particular in that it's usually responsible for generating the arterial stress that is required to perfuse the systemic movement but at the same time has its own perfusion impeded for the duration of the systolic part of the cardiac cycle. Due to the fact that myocardial contraction is closely related to coronary waft and oxygen shipping, stability of oxygen delivery and needs is a crucial determinant of the ordinary beat-to-beat characteristic of the heart. When this dating relationship is acutely disrupted via sicknesses affecting coronary blood waft, the ensuing imbalance can immediately precipitate a different cycle, whereby ischemia-caused contractile dysfunction precipitates hypo-tension and, in addition, myocardial ischemia.

A coronary MI occurs while a coronary artery is blocked unexpectedly as shown in Figure 7.1 or has very slow blood drift. The same original cause of instant blockage in an artery is the development of a blood clot (thrombus).

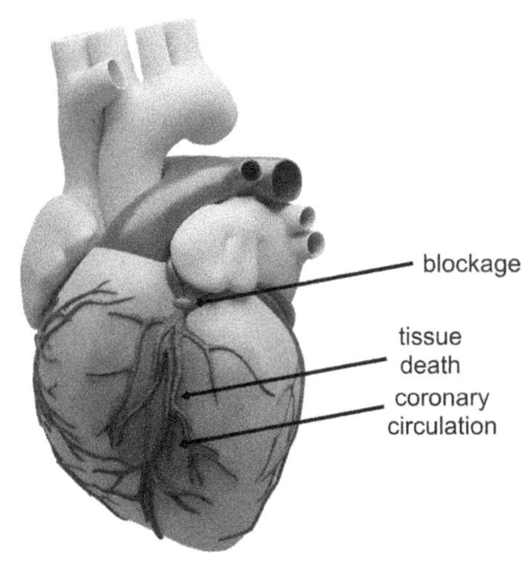

FIGURE 7.1
Myocardial Infarction (MI).

The clotting commonly forms in the interior of an artery that already has been shrunk via atherosclerosis, wherein fats accumulate alongside the inner partitions of vein. The plaque at one end breaks away and forms a clot. The interrupted blood glide can harm or smash part of the heart muscle [2].

7.1.2 Types of MI

There are numerous forms of MI: STEMI (ST segment elevation MI), NSTEMI (Non-STEMI), coronary spasm or unstable angina (present at relaxation) silent coronary heart attack (no chest pain seen, visible in diabetics). Strong angina is precipitated by using physical pressure or exercise like walking or heavy weightlifting, demand ischemia or cardiac arrest (not a heart attack).

7.1.2.1 STEMI (ST-segment elevation myocardial infarction)

A STEMI is a critical form of heart tissue damage in which an artery is completely blocked, and a major portion of the coronary heart muscle is not able to obtain blood. "ST-segment elevation" as shown in Figure 7.3 refers to a shape that indicates on an electrocardiogram (EKG).

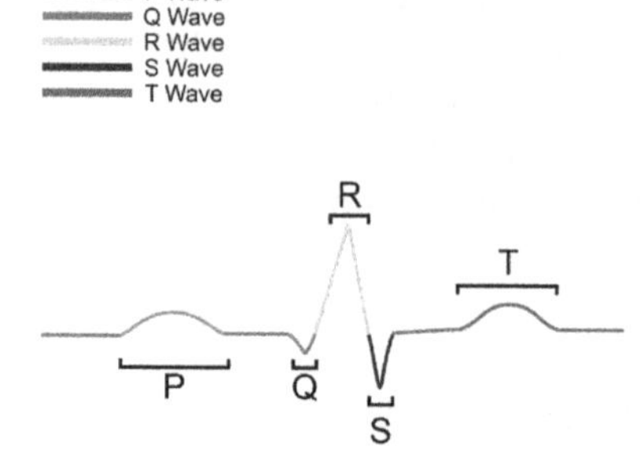

FIGURE 7.2
Normal ECG.

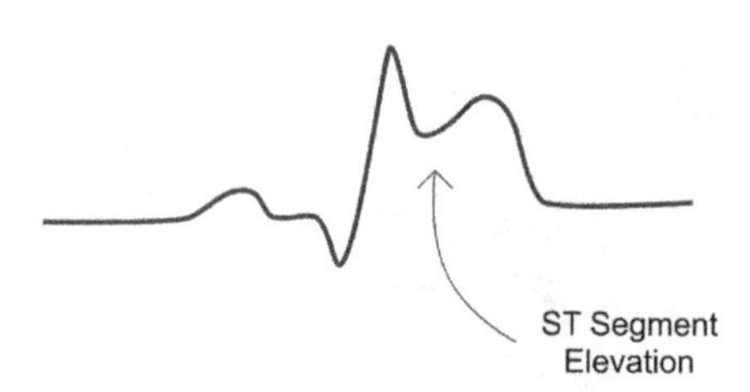

FIGURE 7.3
STEMI.

7.1.2.2 NSTEMI (non-ST segment elevation myocardial infarction)

A NSTEMI is coronary heart tissue damage that does not display a change in ST-segment elevation on an ECG and that results in much less harm to the affected person's heart. But those sufferers will observe a positive for a protein referred to as troponin in their blood, which is revealed in the cardiac muscle when it is damaged. In NSTEMI coronary heart failures, it is very possible that any artery blockages are fragmentary or brief.

7.1.2.3 Angina

Angina is when the artery wall reinforces, and blood passing through the artery is confined – possibly leading to chest pain, or blood flow is interrupt altogether – inflicting heart damage. Artery contraction comes and goes. Due to the fact there might not be a build-up of plaque or a thrombus within the capillary, an artery convulsion might not be located through imaging referred to as an angiogram that is normally done to test capillaries for blockages.

7.1.2.4 Demand Ischemia (DI)

DI is another kind of coronary heart tissue damage for which congestion within the capillaries won't be seen. It takes place just when the affected person's heart desires greater oxygen than is available in the body's delivery system. It can occur in patients with contamination, anemia, or Tachyarrhythmia (atypical speedy heart rate). Blood reports will show the presence of enzymes that indicate harm to the heart tissues.

7.1.2.5 Cardiac Arrest

Cardiopulmonary arrest is brought about when the heart's electric system breaks down. The heart stops beating correctly. Therefore, the coronary heart's pumping function is arrested.

A stroke can quickly result in the person's demise if the right steps aren't taken immediately. This paralysis of the heart can be reversed if CPR (cardiopulmonary resuscitation) is done and a defibrillator is used to shock the coronary heart and restore a regular heart rhythm inside a few moments.

Those other motives encompass electrolyte disturbances, which include low or high potassium or low magnesium, congenital abnormalities, or severe pumping characteristics of the heart [3].

The above discussion is how the heart works within the human frame. However, there are various elements that should be taken into consideration: Many studies are proposed in myocardial infarction. It is, additionally, essential to recognize all MI information that has been proposed by doctors and researchers. Numerous once-unknown factors have been discovered in research about MI. Those research efforts aren't associated with AI/ML, and to date no technique has been proposed to detect early MI.

The major drawback of these researches is that they mainly focus on the implementation of classification technique for MI prognosis, rather than considering various data-cleaning and pruning techniques that make a dataset acceptable and also responsible to increase the accuracy of the prediction.

Other drawback is myocardial infarction detection is not done under the guidance of doctors and also does not used recent medical experiences. They only know the actual cause of MI nowadays, and various parameters are changing due to humanity's more stressful life.

7.2 Literature Review

7.2.1 Clinical Investigations

There are various discussions and investigations on medical diseases in various papers that are discussed here.

Patients with tachycardia have weakened practical capability and diminished quality of life. Low-load blood flow restricting resistance exercise (BFRRE) may want to enhance functional potential and promote making best of circumstances in sufferers with coronary heart failure (CHF). However, blood flow restricted resistance exercise (BFRRE), not remote ischemic conditioning (RIC), improves useful potential quality of life [4].

Individuals living in neighborhoods where walks are not possible seem to be physically inactive and much more prone to advanced hypertension, obesity and diabetes mellitus. It's doubtful whether a neighborhood's walkability is a threat to the future of one's cardiorespiratory ailments. Adults living in less walkable neighborhoods had a higher ten-year acute MI disorder threat than those dwelling in walkable neighborhoods [5].

Little is understood about the approximate length of the time period trends in consequence of sufferers with ischemic stroke in China to assess longitudinal trends in those results during the last 15 years and to discover possible elements behind the trends. There have been encouraging declines in the chances of incapacity and death at 3 and 12 months after ischemic stroke in the Chinese language-cohort studied in 2002 and 2016 [6].

In heart failure (HF), the three fundamental steps of cardiac strength metabolism are as follows: substrate uptake, oxidative phosphorylation and shuffling of strength from mitochondria to the cytosol [7].

The prevalence of thyroid dysfunction and associations with cardiovascular outcomes encompasses a huge, expected cohort of outpatients with pre-present coronary heart failure [8].

MI is a main reason of maternal illness and mortality. Heart failure (HF) occurrence, correlates, and consequences among maternity hospitalizations amongst females thirteen to 49 years of age become identified. MI is associated with rising chances of maternal illness and deaths. At some point of the hospitalization, mothers with excessive-risk have to be diagnosed and an intelligence system developed before discharge [9].

The patients admitted to hospitals with new appearance or aggravated symptoms of MI with preserved ejection fraction (HFpEF) face an excessive risk of death, with about one-third of the sufferers dying within 12 months [10].

Nonpulsatile pulmonary blood drift in Fontan affects results in pulmonary vascular sickness [11].

The ketone frame oxidation expands in tachycardia, and elevated ketone frame utilization decreases oxidative pressure and guards against coronary heart failure [12].

Family records and age are also a very vital issues because of the risk of MI. After 59 years of age there is much less improvement in fitness. So, it must be concluded that age is likewise an important issue for MI [13].

Sadness is three times as frequent in patients after a cardiac attack than in the main population. Unhappiness after a coronary heart attack is problematic on account of the accompanying misery and life struggle. Also, it obviously increases one's chance of having other coronary heart attacks or dying over the ensuing months and years.

Numerous traits that are discovered in depressed people might account for poor prospects after a coronary heart attack are:

- ✓ No longer taking medicinal drugs as prescribed.
- ✓ Continuing to smoke.
- ✓ Much less physical interest.
- ✓ Accelerated stress hormone ranges.
- ✓ Extended blood sugar and lipid degrees.
- ✓ Increased tendency of blood to clot.
- ✓ Increased inflammatory cytokine ranges criteria for predominant depressive disorder.
- ✓ Depressed temperament.
- ✓ Markedly diminished interest or delight in almost all activities most of the day; extreme weight loss, or urge for food.
- ✓ Insomnia or hypersomnia.
- ✓ Psychomotor agitation or retardation.
- ✓ Fatigue and feelings of guilt.
- ✓ Dwindled capacity to think or listen; indecisiveness.
- ✓ Recurrent thoughts of dying, suicidal ideation [14].

Any other parameter, such as the excessive presentation of diabetic symptoms ought to anticipate the threat of further coronary events [15].

It would be evident, then, to study cardiac ischemia at the single-cell level. There is cause to suspect that this latest technique will reinstate the field of single-cell ischemia research. This will create an insistence for developments in the basic chemical measurements of single cells [16].

Various preventions for coronary heart attack and stroke are: [17]

- ✓ Stop smoking.
- ✓ Engage in physical activity.
- ✓ Find diet remedies.
- ✓ Preserve/reduce weight.
- ✓ Manage blood pressure.
- ✓ Establish LDL cholesterol control/statin remedy.
- ✓ Manage blood sugar.
- ✓ Limit alcohol consumption.
- ✓ Take aspirin as recommended.

Early signs and symptoms of an MI. Who's at risk?

In males, the danger of coronary heart assault increases appreciably after the age of 45. In females, MI are much more expected to arise in the years after menopause (generally, in their fifties). It can be that younger people also may have MI. Other than age, elements that increase the hazard for coronary heart attack are diabetes mellitus, obesity and so forth. Those who have one or more of these factors should see their doctor to learn how to lessen your risk of heart attack [18].

Coronary disease caution symptoms?

1. Chest pain.
2. Pain in different areas of the upper frame.
3. Shortness of breath.
4. Women and men with a family record of coronary heart attacks should avoid smoking [19].

The family records of MI can be a beneficial aid for finding younger men with high-risk for coronary disease [20].

The possibility of a coronary heart attack in the morning is increased and possibly more severe around 6 a.m., and midday is associated with the maximum harm. Heart attack severity was calculated by way of examining top concentrations of creatine kinase(ck) and troponin-i, key enzymes launched in response to muscle injury. High blood pressure is the main cause of for coronary heart attack and stroke [21].

7.2.2 Healthcare and Artificial Intelligence

Era of black box magic has come into the picture, that is, artificial intelligence (AI), which has made a great impact on every area of research as well as in medical diagnosis. A lot of work is in progress to develop a model that should diagnosed early to save a human life. There are many diseases that are not curable if timely action is not taken. The mortality rate of cancer and myocardial infarction (MI) are very high nowadays. Heart diseases cause 32 million deaths per year worldwide. Every 33 seconds someone dies from heart disease worldwide. Research work with AI proposed in medical fields is remarkable.

Hierarchical Temporal Memory Algorithm (HTM) is a real-time anomaly detection algorithm. For the present chapter, HTM has been implemented and tested on ECG datasets in order to detect cardiac anomalies. Experiments showed good performance in terms of specificity, sensitivity and execution time [22].

Data mining, as a solution to extricate a hidden sample from the clinical dataset, is implemented to a database in this research. All the algorithms in class approach differentiate from every other to obtain better accuracy. Similarly, for growth and the correctness of the solution, the dataset is preprocessed with the aid of various supervised and unsupervised algorithms. The two essential duties that can be wished to improve the classifier come under the category data mining, and those are clustering and classification. In k-means clustering, the start-point choice affects the outcomes of the algorithm, each in the number of clusters located and their centers. Techniques to increase the k-approach clustering set of rules are mentioned. With the assist of these strategies' efficiency, accuracy and overall performance are advanced. So, to enhance the performance of clusters, the normalization that is a pre-processing stage is used to decorate the Euclidean distance by calculating extra closer centers, which in the end results in a discounted quantity of iterations, a good way to reduce the computational time in comparison to k-means clustering. Eventually, the classifiers are advanced with logistic regression by the usage of the records extracted by means of k-means clustering. The methods adopted inside the design of classifier show tremendously in phrases of type consequences greater in comparison to clustering techniques. This research proved that normalization of parameters improved accuracy [23].

In this chapter four different classifiers were compared, with the conclusion that the LAD (Logical Analysis of Data) tree has minimum mean absolute and relative absolute errors. The four are Bayesian network, DT (Decision Tree), LAD tree and J48 tree [24].

In this research, 53 papers were reviewed, originally published between 2008 and 2017, focusing on EMG, EEG, ECG, and EOG. For big and varied datasets, Deep learning performed better than classic analysis and ML [25].

The inspiration for this chapter turned into developing effective therapeutics with the use of information-mining techniques that can assist in remedying situations. In addition to information mining, types of algorithms like DT, NN, Bayesian classifier (BC), SVM, association rule, k- nearest neighbor category are used to diagnosis heart disease. Among those algorithms, support vector system (SVM) gave an excellent end result [26].

The alternating decision tree is a novel type of classification rule. It is a generalization that decision trees are combinations of voted decision stumps and voted decision trees. Researchers applied this approach to MI patient data collected from numerous hospitals in Hyderabad. Optimization of features improved the competence of the learning algorithm. They used principal component analysis to determine the necessary features of MI data. Exploratory results have shown that their decision support system achieved better accuracy and proved its usefulness in the prognosis of MI [27].

Exceptional statistics mining and neural network class technology were used in analyzing the risk of tachycardia happening based on hazard factors. The risk level of something is classifying the usage of techniques like k-nearest neighbor set of rules, decision trees, genetic algorithm, Naïve Bayes and so forth, and the accuracy becomes extreme when using greater attributes and combinations of above strategies. It was additionally cautioned that combinations of sets of rules improve accuracy [28].

The authors reviewed the challenges in the analysis of heart ailments using an EKG signal and the latest traits inside the approach analysis of the ST-segment on an EKG signal through supplying the EKG signal pre-processing, feature extraction and classification techniques. This revealed confirmed diverse modifications determined in the EKG signal because of blockage of coronary arteries [29].

An exhaustive survey that mining required information from the medical data helped us to support well-informed diagnoses and decisions [30].

This chapter features remote sensing inputs of the human body that consisted of pulse rate and temperature. The inputs that had been used for sensing and tracking can ship the records via wi-fi sensors. The sensing records would be consistently accumulated in a database and might be used for telling the affected person about any hidden problems and give a feasible prognosis. An advanced machine that quantifies human heartbeats and body temperature of the affected person sends the statistics to the consumer or server stop via the usage of a microcontroller at a reasonable cost and with wonderful effect [31].

This research aimed to conclude some of the recent work on diagnosis of cardiac diseases using data mining techniques, exploration with the various combinations of mining algorithms used and presumptions about which technique(s) are effectual and coherent [32].

This chapter summarizes the various techniques that use echocardiography (EKG) for the prognosis and examination of mitral valve disorders at the advance stages and lessens the death rate of cardiac attack diseases. This chapter summarizes the advantages over the manual and computerized methods, and the assessment of performance is studied more accurately. By this survey, the authors culminate with the proximal flow convergence method that gave better results in contrast with other methods and techniques [33].

In this chapter, they present a review report on patients suffering from MI by literature survey, which measured the Electrocardiogram (ECG), body temperature and pulse rate of users through the sensors. The main advantage of this device is to show results on android mobile phones with percentage values, which makes it comfortable for patients to see their own health readings for early and prompt management of any imminent cardiac disease [34].

Many wi-fi communique technologies are advanced for heart-condition diagnosis. Data mining algorithms are very helpful in the prognosis and analysis of an MI. This survey is administered on various single and hybrid facts processing algorithms if we want to spot the set of rules that most correctly suits the central disorder prediction with an extreme level of accuracy. A survey is carried out on diverse information mining strategies helpful for the diagnosis and analysis of cardiac ailments. The authors proposed several algorithms, but there are certain obstacles to those algorithms such as the artificial neural (ANN) community carried out nicely, most effective with the linear dataset, the overall performance of decision tree set of rules becomes negative with a big quantity of datasets. [35].

This chapter supplied a review on two different complicated illnesses, which include cardiac disease and most cancer disorders, and firmly found the triumphing literature work searching for out-sizeable understanding in this vicinity and summed up specific tactics used in ailment diagnosing. The selection of data mining approaches isn't always the same for all. It honestly relies upon on the dataset type: if the dataset is labelled then the best method is to use classification algorithms even as in case of unlabeled dataset, it is far better to use a clustering technique that's exceptionally suitable for pattern recognition [36].

In this research two models were developed: the first was to filter those parameters that are more responsible for MI, and another model was to predict MI. Accuracy of the model was 70 percent. A 2012 dataset was used for this model [37].

The research supplied a top-level view of ECG denoising techniques alongside feature extraction and recognition strategies used for heartbeat classification and myocardial infarction detection. It was observed that the recorded ECG signal may comprise specific forms of artifacts that ought to be eliminated before further processing. Based on this observation, it has been discovered that baseline wandering, electricity line interferences and electromyographic noises are successfully eliminated with the aid of wavelet-based techniques [38].

This research provided an expeditious and facile review and interpretation of available prediction models using data mining from 2004 to 2016. The collation has shown the accuracy level of each model given by various researchers. It is noted that all the techniques available have not used big data analytics. Use of big data analytics along with data mining will give encouraging results to get the best precision in designing the prediction model [39].

A survey of diverse denoising tactics that have come up over recent years has been offered in this chapter. FIR and IIR filtering, low and high-frequency noise removal strategies, Quadrature filtering, adaptive noise cancellation strategies, non-local means denoising strategies (NLM), empirical mode decomposition (EMD), variational mode decomposition (VMD), wavelet transform denoising strategies and up-to-date traits are mentioned along comparatives studies. Threshold selection also has an extraordinary effect on the results. All these methods are applied on the ECG signal to achieve a better-denoised signal, and the exceptional method amidst them may be observed only when combos of all available techniques are tested for the system with distinct thresholds and inputs [40].

Patients with peripheral artery disease (PAD) are at high risk of acute limb ischemia (ALI), a morbid event which will end in limb loss. They investigated the causes, sequelae, and predictors of ALI during a contemporary population with symptomatic PAD and whether protease-activated receptor 1 antagonism with vorapaxar reduced ALI overall and by type. It was concluded that patients with symptomatic PAD are at a high risk of ALI, facing a risk similar to that of stroke or MI [41].

Consistent with the analysis mode, it is apparent that many of authors use numerous technologies and exceptional variety of attributes for their observation. Hence, one-of-a-kind technology gave unique precision, relying on some of the attributes considered. Using the KNN and ID3 algorithm, the risk rate of coronary heart condition was detected and, consequently, the accuracy stage also provided for numerous attributes. In future, the numbers of attributes will be reduced, and accuracy might multiply the usage of some other algorithms [42].

The authors proposed a replacement approach to detect the state of affairs of MI from nearby wall warping, which has a cost for prospect stratification from recurring inspection, like (3D) echocardiography. The channel combines a non-linear dimensionality discount of contortion styles and two multi-scale kernel regressions. Confidence in the diagnosis is assessed by a map of local uncertainties, which integrates plausible infarct locations generated from the space of reduced dimensionality [43].

Adults with eczema are more inclined to smoke cigarettes, consume alcohol, and have an inactive lifestyle. The authors sought to work out whether adult eczema is related to increased cardiovascular and cerebrovascular disease.

And that they found that adults with atopic eczema may have increased disorders, attacks and stroke. Eczema is additionally a crucial factor for MI [44].

The research discussed the problems intrinsic to electrocardiogram (ECG) classification and presented an in-depth survey of pre-processing techniques, ECG databases, feature extraction techniques, ANN-based classifiers and performance measures to deal with the introduced issues. The survey also presented an in-depth analysis of input beat selection and output of the classifiers. However, it is noticed from the survey that neural networks are good candidates for ECG classification in terms of classification accuracy on training and testing datasets [45].

7.3 Research Gap

After in-depth analysis of the research and also with detailed discussion with the doctors, specialist in myocardial infarction (MI), we found the followings gaps where the researchers have not yet contributed for accurate and early diagnosis of myocardial infarction (MI).

Previous work has been done on traditional risk factors/parameters that are already responsible for MI referred by cardiologists, that is, mostly high blood pressure (BP), cholesterol, ECG and so forth. This is also used in medical sciences where doctors are using the same traditional way to detect MI in patients. There is a gap between research work and doctors' diagnosis due to lack of considering parameters of those patients who have already been diagnosed with MI and are changed according to lifestyle, eating habits and so forth. The increase in cases of MI means that there are chances of some new factors that are more vulnerable for MI and not considered. It is also found that the researchers have not considered doctors' lifetime experiences to diagnose and enhance the accuracy of the model. Nowadays the perspective of life of humans has changed, and the lifestyle, eating habits, work stress and so forth are responsible factors for MI.

The previous research is based on post myocardial infarction diagnosis. It is necessary in today's environment to detect the early possibility of MI. There is a need of research work to be carried out on an existing model to increase the efficiency and accuracy of the model by gathering recent responsible parameters of MI rather than relying on existing ones.

There is a scope of working on those models that use only classification techniques. They have not considered pruning and cleaning techniques that increase the accuracy. Normalized parameters are needed to feed the model to get efficient and accurate detection of MI early.

7.3.1 Research Objectives

- To survey additional parameters that lead to myocardial infarction.
- To develop an intelligent framework and a machine learning (ML) model for accurate diagnosis of MI.
- Creating the dataset from the patient's records.
- Improve the feature extraction method with additional parameters.
- Improve the Support Vector Machine with additional parameters.
- To prepare dataset with new risk factors of MI.
- To prepare the dataset with patient history.
- To prepare a machine learning model with new dataset for early detection of MI.
- To train and test the model for early detection of MI.
- To verify and validate proposed data-mining model using a case study and with actual patient data.
- To validate model by giving input of patients through doctors and cardiologists.

7.4 Proposed Methods

(a) Schematic Diagram of Proposed System

The requirement and realization are that without access to medical records and lab data there were limits to making accurate diagnoses. Diagnosis relies upon many different types of (accurate) data, from patient history to physical examination to lab data to past medical records and to radiographic findings. Each patient's immune system and history are different.

It is very important to note that if early prediction is possible then the mortality rate with MI will definitely lessen and the lives of people will be up graded. The most important thing is to consider those parameters of MI that are not included in early research but are most vulnerable for MI in life today.

There is always a perspective to stepping out from existing approach and exploring beyond the limits of other's findings. Therefore, there is a need for designing a model that will predict MI early, based on the parameters fed to the model. In order to enhance the accuracy of the prognosis of MI for clinicians and clinical scientists, the input in our system is gathered from many doctors personally and the patient's data through proper channels with history of MI, and this dataset is given to the predictive model, which then verifies and validates the proposed model as shown in Figure 7.4. Early detection of MI will save many lives. This system will be helpful to doctors' assistants and nurses to take timely action if a doctor is not available in the hospital.

(b) Block Diagram of Proposed Model

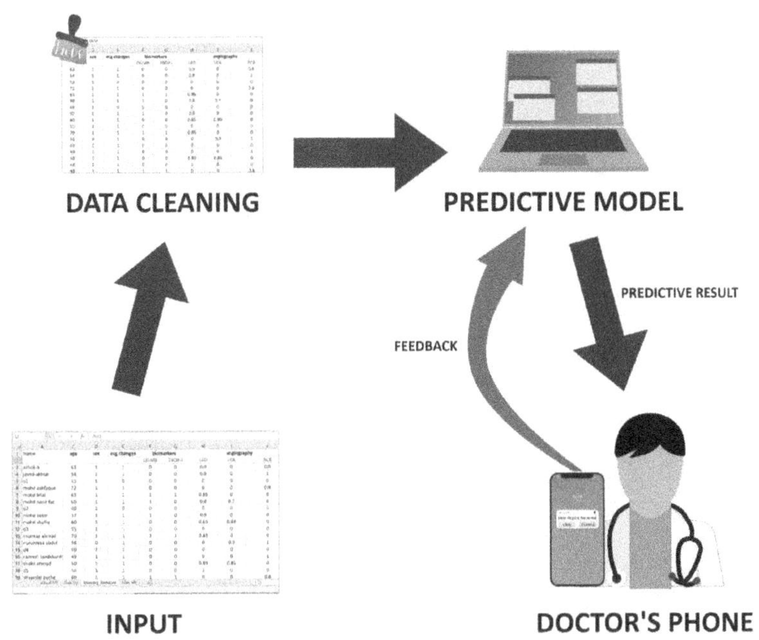

FIGURE 7.4
Schematic Diagram of Predictive Model.

7.4.1 Bucketization

Here, machine learning algorithms are used to enhance the accuracy of the model for detection of myocardial infarction (MI). Some features might have sub-features. The parameters needed to detect the MI are not necessarily in the same format or categorical data, that must be converted into separate numerical data using bucketization method, and it is useful to organize the input data into different buckets so that the system will read datasets properly.

So, bucketization is used to make buckets for sub-features by breaking down the main features into sub-features.

In our dataset, angiography, chest pain type and blood pressure features have sub-features. Those are considered separate features and included in the dataset. One more feature having three values: early MI (Angina), MI and non-MI, which are bucketized (refer to Figure 7.5).

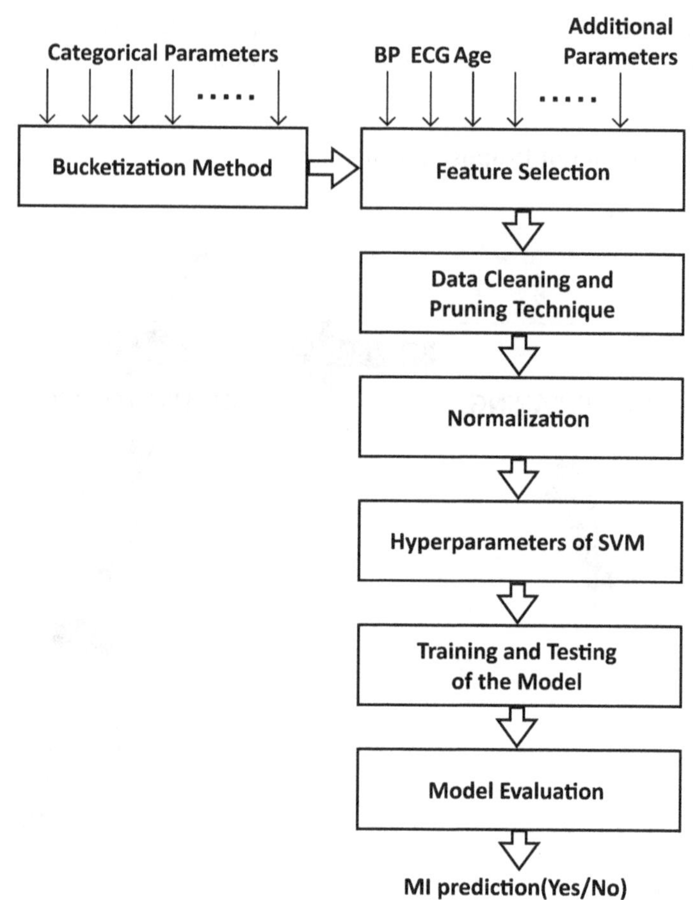

FIGURE 7.5
Block Diagram of Proposed Model.

7.4.2 Feature Selection Techniques

Feature selection is important to enhance the accuracy of the model by eliminating irrelevant attributes that are not participating in the prediction [46]. Selecting optimal features to train the model is always good practice to achieve the objective of the model and also useful to increase the accuracy of the model. Here, subsets of features are obtained through feature selection techniques and given to the model for training purposes. Due to this feature selection, the accuracy of the model is enhanced.

In our research, we gathered the important features by literature review. After that, a survey was done on those features, and opinion of experts was considered in order to eliminate unwanted attributes.

There are various techniques of feature selection.

7.4.2.1 Filter Method

This method is used to check the relevance of the attribute with the goal attribute, checking the correlation between input data and target attribute. If any characteristic is affecting the objective's attribute then that attribute is taken into consideration as a relevant characteristic. This means there is some correlation and dependency of the goal attribute with this characteristic. Here every attribute is compared with goal characteristics and checked whether the target characteristic is being affected or not. Any irrelevant attribute that isn't always affecting the target attribute is eliminated. Numerous techniques are used for this reason, such as:

- Chi-Square Test: In preferred terms, this approach is used to test the independence of events. This test only assesses associations between categorical variables and does not make any inferences about causation.
- Variance Threshold: This technique of attribute selection gets rid of all capabilities whose variance no longer meets a few thresholds. Typically, it eliminates all the zero-variance attributes, which means all of the attributes that have the similar value in all samples.
- Information Gain: Information gain or IG measures how much information an attribute provides about the class. Therefore, we can focus on which attribute in a given set of training feature is the most significant for discerning between the classes to be learned (refer to Figure 7.6).

7.4.2.2 Wrapper Method

Multiple models are created in this method by using different subsets of features with the target attribute. Each model's accuracy and error rate are checked, and, those model's features are considered in the model that gives best accuracy. However, this method requires high computation. It becomes increasingly expensive the larger the number of features.

- Genetic algorithms (GA): This can be used to find a subset of attributes. CHCGA is the amend model of this set of rules, which converges quicker and provides an extra effective search, preserving variety and keeping away from the status of the population.

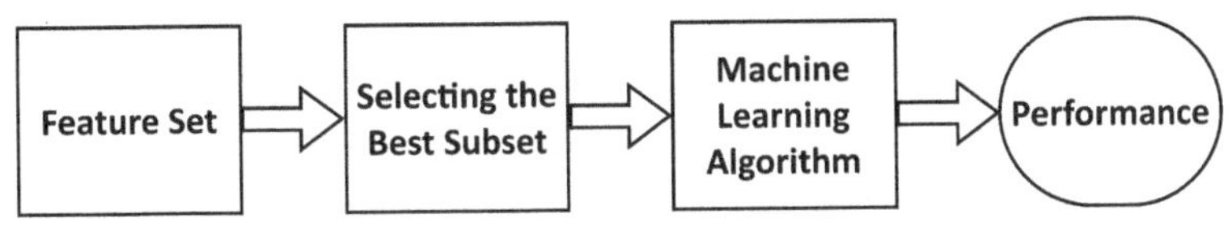

FIGURE 7.6
Block Diagram of Filter Method.

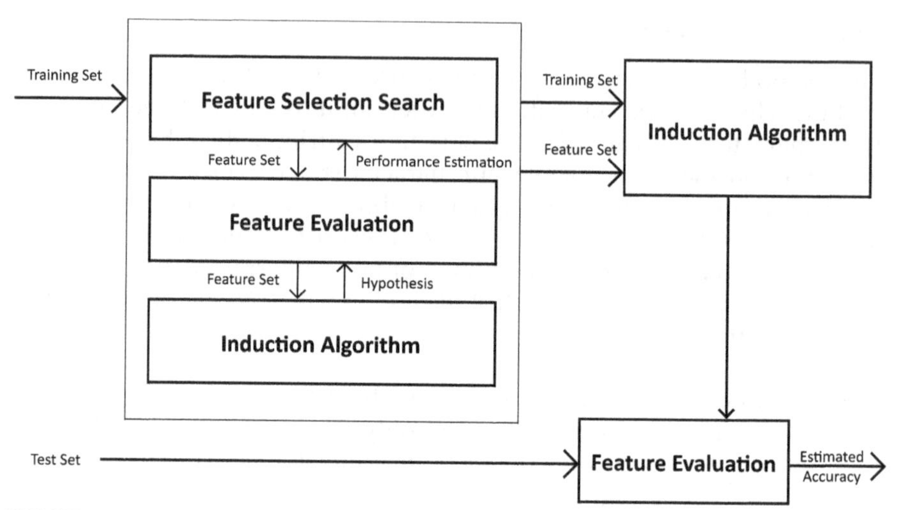

FIGURE 7.7
Block Diagram of Wrapper Method.

- Recursive feature elimination: RFE is a feature selection technique which lays out the model and eliminates the incapacitated attribute until the specified number of attributes are satisfied. Here, the attributes are classified by the model's coefficient or feature-importance attributes.
- Sequential feature selection: This naive algorithm starts with a null set and then adds one attribute to the first step, which shows the greater value for the objective function, and from the second step onwards the remaining attributes are added one by one to the current subset and thus the new subset is appraised. This process is repeated until the essential count of features is included (refer to Figure 7.7).

7.4.2.3 Embedded Method

This approach is used to locate the usefulness of characteristic. It works almost similar to the wrapper technique. The simplest distinction among these two is that it requires much less computation in comparison to the wrapper approach. Capacity of overfitting is much less as compared to the wrapper approach. This method combines the effectiveness of both the preceding methods and performs the selection of variables within the process of schooling and is typically particular to gaining knowledge of machines. This approach essentially learns which feature gives the utmost to the precision of the model.

- L1 regularization method inclusive of LASSO: Least absolute shrinkage and selection operator, this is a linear model that calculates the sparse coefficients and is helpful in a few conditions due to its tendency to prefer solutions with fewer parameter values.

- Ridge regression (L2 Regularization): L2 regularization is likewise referred to as ridge regression or Tikhonov Regularization, which solves a regression model wherein the loss function is the linear least-squares characteristic and regularization.
- Elastic net: This linear regression version is educated with L1 and L2 as regularizing, which allows for mastering a sparse model where few of the weights are non-zero, like LASSO, and alternatively keeping the regularization properties of ridge regression.

Attributes selection is the approach of decreasing data dimensionality even while doing predictive analysis. One important cause is that machine learning follows the rule of thumb: "garbage in, garbage out." This is why one needs to be very worried about the data that is being provided to the model. Feature selection is used to simply accept the selected capabilities of the input parameter as many undesirable attributes may avoid performance.

Function selection strategies simplify the model's getting to know styles to be able to make it simpler to interpret via the researchers. It especially gets rid of the results of the curse of dimensionality. Aside from, this method reduces the trouble of overfitting with the aid of improving the generalization inside the model. As a consequence, it enables better information of data, improves the prognosis of overall performance, lowering the computational time in addition to space that is needed to run the algorithm.

7.4.3 Data Cleaning and Pruning Technique

Data cleaning and pruning technique is performed on the selected data so that a correctly cleaned and pruned dataset provides much better precision than an unclean one with missing values. Data cleaning is the process of preparing data for analysis by removing or modifying data that is incorrect, incomplete, unrelated, redundant or improperly formatted.

Steps involved in data cleaning are:

(a) **Removal of Unwanted Observations**
This includes deleting duplicate/redundant or irrelevant values from the dataset.

(b) **Fixing Structural Errors**
The errors that arise during measurement, transfer of data or other similar situations are called structural errors.

(c) **Managing Unwanted Outliers:** Outliers can cause problems with certain type of model. These outliers generate two types or errors, that is, data-processing errors and sampling errors.

(d) **Handling Missing Data:** Here, first observe the data and see how many missing points we have. Figure out why the data is missing and fill in missing values.

In our datasets, some information about the patients were missing, but those values cannot be filled in with assumptions. So, those missing values were filled with the help of expertise.

There are various methods for data cleaning, such as:

- Parsing
- Correcting
- Matching
- Consolidation
- Dealing with missing data
- Dealing with Incorrect & noisy date

Pruning is used in the decision tree to reduce or minimize classification errors.

Outlier cleaning is required if input parameters gathered during the survey are rare in diagnosing MI.

Forward fill and backward method: predictive mean matching (PMM), interpolation method will be adopted in the research if the data collected during the survey has missing values.

Missing values functions are applied on existing datasets. In our dataset it is not advisable to fill values with missing values without the involvement of experts. So here we cautiously discussed matters with the experts about the missing values (refer to Figure 7.8).

7.4.4 Normalization

Normalization is a scaling technique or a mapping technique or a pre-processing stage, where we find new range from an existing range. It is useful to make data in the same units.

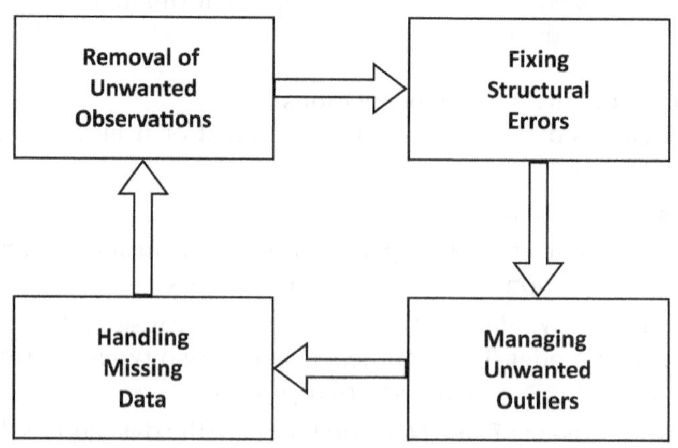

FIGURE 7.8
Block Diagram of Data Cleaning Technique.

It is helpful for the prediction. There are some existing normalization techniques, namely Min-Max, Z score and Decimal scaling. An improvised version of normalization technique has been used in this research with an additional focus on fuzzy based normalization methods.

The standardization method uses this formula:

$$z = (x-u)/s$$

Where z is the new value, x is the original value, u is the mean and s is the standard deviation as shown in above equation. In our research the maximum range of high blood pressure for MI patients and angiography parameters and so forth are scaled as a result of discussions of experts.

7.4.5 Machine Learning

Machine learning is useful when specialists are unable to give an explanation for their expertise while human information does not exist.

In machine learning:

- All problems are data; all solutions are capabilities/maps.
- Cognitive Task-Human beings get sensory inputs as qualia (qualitative inputs). We have to convert those qualitative inputs into numbers, that is, input vectors. Similarly, outputs that people give also need to be transformed into numbers, that is, output or goal vectors.
- Determining suitable inputs and outputs for mastering the system is critical and challenging part of the process.

7.5 Experimental Result with Existing Dataset

It has been discovered that the dataset accessible on Kaggle is from 1989. There are 76 attributes, but a dataset of 14 attributes is given. Four of them are concerned with MI diagnosis. All input features are numerically valued. The data was gathered from the following four locations:

1. Cleveland.data
2. Hungarian.data
3. Long-beach-va.data
4. Switzerland.data

Each database has the same number of attributes. Datasets have 76 raw attributes, but only 14 of them are actually used, as mention in Table 7.1.

TABLE 7.1

List of Attributes

Sr. No.	Attribute Name
1.	age
2.	sex
3.	Cp (chest pain type) 1: typical angina 2: atypical angina 3: non-anginal pain 4: asymptomatic
4.	restbps (resting blood pressure (in mm Hg on admission to the hospital)
5.	chol (serum cholesterol in mg/dl)
6.	fbs (fasting blood sugar > 120 mg/dl) (1 = true; 0 = false)
7.	restecg (resting electrocardiographic results) 0: normal 1: having ST-T wave abnormality (T wave inversions and/or STelevation or depression of > 0.05 mV) 2: showing probable or definite left ventricular hypertrophy by Estes' criteria
8.	thalach (maximum heart rate achieved)
9.	exang (exercise induced angina (1 = yes; 0 = no)
10.	oldpeak (ST depression induced by exercise relative to rest)
11.	slope (the slope of the peak exercise ST segment) 1: upsloping 2: flat 3: down sloping
12.	Ca (number of major vessels (0–3) colored by fluoroscopy)
13.	thal (3 = normal; 6 = fixed defect; 7 = reversable defect)
14.	num (the predicted attribute) diagnosis of heart disease (angiographic disease status) 0: < 50% diameter narrowing 1: > 50% diameter narrowing

(a) **NAN (Not a Number) Analysis:** In this analysis, the various datasets of the countries are compared with missing values. It is observed that the dataset of Cleveland has a minimum of missing values as shown in the following graph: Figure 7.9 (a–d).

(b) **Various Machine Learning Algorithms Used on Merged Dataset**

Table 7.2 below includes a comparative look at the various algorithms. In this study, four datasets from Cleveland and three other places are merged, as the attributes are same. Data processing is applied to fill NaN (not a number) values and are filled with mean values. As the dataset has a number of rows, it therefore seems the result shown is very accurate. However, such a diagnosis for a deadly disease related to the heart cannot be trusted upon since the given diagnosis is not proper. This gap can be filled only with the consultation of experts. Hence, this gap is likewise taken into consideration within the studies.

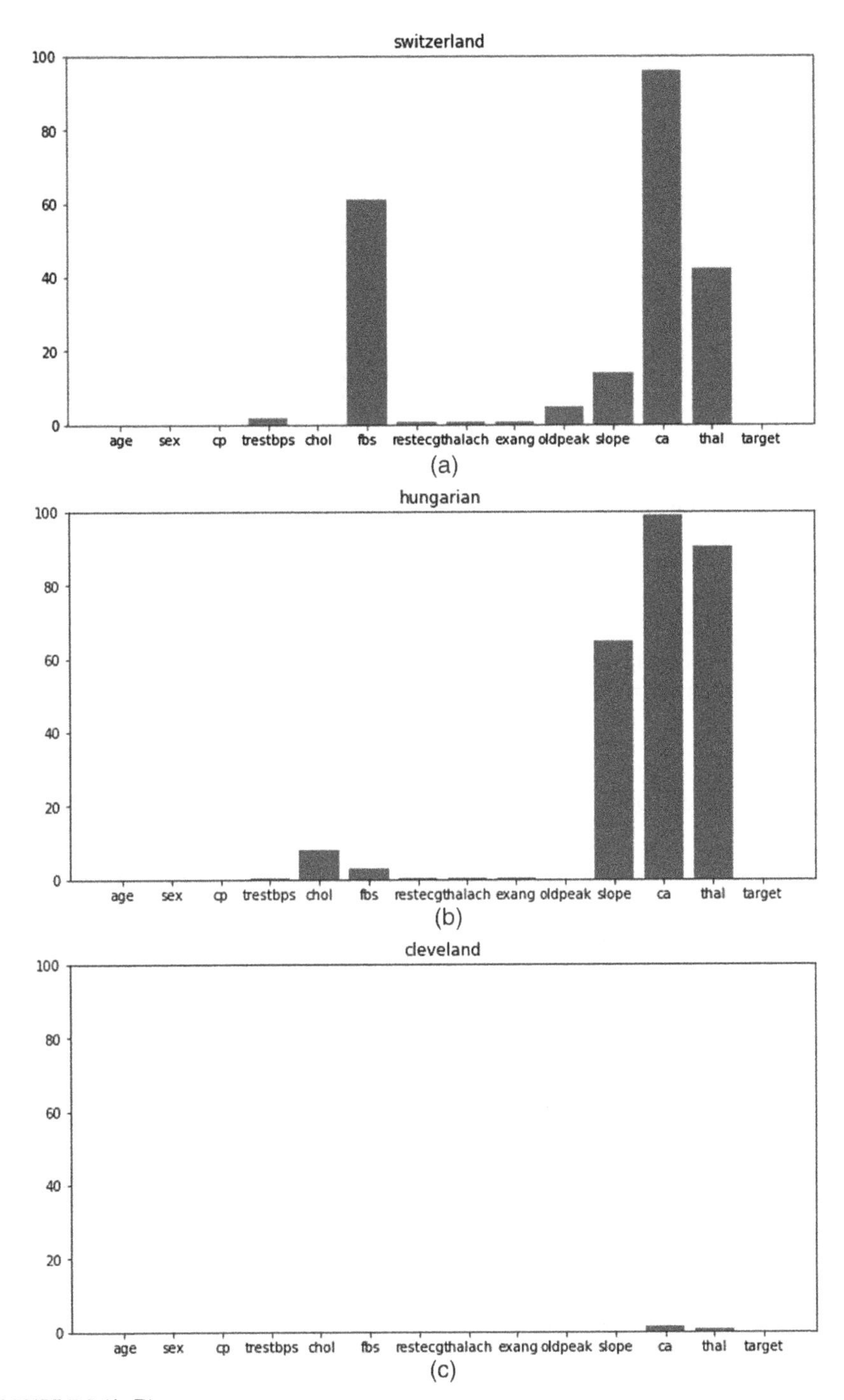

FIGURE 7.9 (A–D)
Graphical Representations of Missing Values of Datasets.

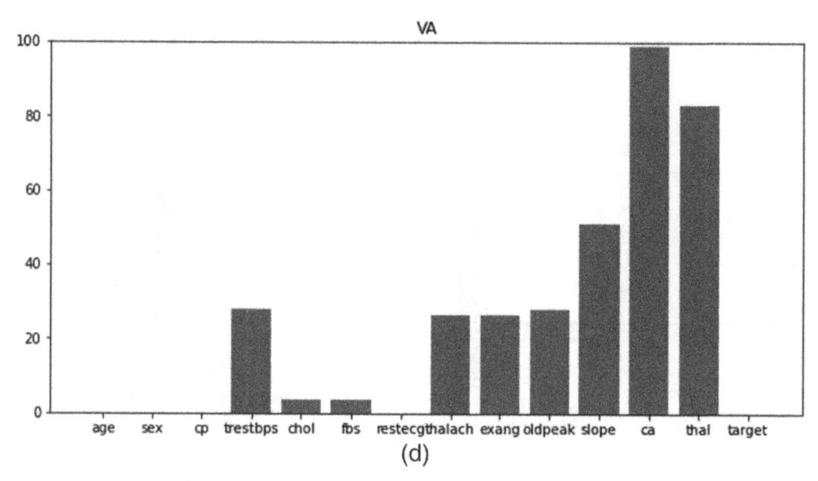

FIGURE 7.9 (A–D) Continued
Graphical Representations of Missing Values of Datasets.

TABLE 7.2
Comparison of Algorithms

Algorithms	Training Set (%)	Testing Set (%)
SVM	100.0	97.82
NAÏVE BAYES	98.36	98.36
LOGISTIC REGRESSION	100.0	100.0
DECISION TREE	100.0	100.0
RANDOM FOREST	100.0	100.0

The model is overfitting because:
Learning that a tree classifies the training data perfectly may not lead to the tree with the best generalization performance.

- There may be noise in the training data
- It may be based on insufficient data

A hypothesis "h" is said to overfit the training data if there is another hypothesis "h`"
Such that,

"h`" has more error than "h" on training data,
"h`" has less error than "h" on test data.

In the above model we have too many missing values that are filled with mean values. Here the model is overfitting due to a smaller amount of

TABLE 7.3

Cleveland Dataset

Algorithms	Training Set (%)	Testing Set (%)
SVM	92.56	80.32
NAÏVE BAYES	86.77	78.68
LOGISTIC REGRESSION	86.36	80.32
DECISION TREE	100.0	75.4
RANDOM FOREST	99.17	75.40

information available. So underfitting occurs when the model is too simple, and overfitting occurs when the model is too complex.

(c) Various Machine Learning Algorithms Used on Cleveland Dataset

After plotting the graph on various datasets of different places as shown in Figure 7.9 (a-d), it is observed that the Cleveland dataset has lowest missing values. Hence it is used for application in machine learning algorithms. Next, algorithms like SVM, Naïve Bayes, Logistic Regression and Random Forest are applied on the dataset. The dataset is then divided into 80:20 ratio, out of which 80 percent of the dataset is considered as training set and 20 percent as testing set. Table 7.3 shows comparison of different algorithms used, resulting in a conclusion that SVM has the highest accuracy.

7.6 Implementation

7.6.1 Survey

A survey has been conducted to assemble data from expertise and patients' reports from various hospitals to produce datasets for detection of myocardial infarction, information from which is transformed into knowledge base.

Step A: Scrutinized Parameters for MI

With diligent study and already-available information from previous researches, attributes listed below are of much importance for MI.

1. Age.
2. High frequency of diabetes.
3. Cigarette smoking.
4. Overweight.
5. Lethargy.

6. Family history of early heart disease.
7. Previous heart disease (PHF).
8. Depression is three times more common in patients after an MI than in the general population.
9. Ketone body oxidation increases MI, and increased ketone body utilization decreases oxidative stress and protects against heart failure.
10. Non-pulsatile pulmonary blood flow in Fontan circulation results in pulmonary vascular disease.
11. The HF with preserved ejection fraction (HFpEF) faces a high risk of death.
12. HF is related with increased risk of maternal mortality and morbidities.
13. Thyroid dysfunction.
14. In heart failure (HF), cardiac energy metabolism is deranged.
15. Proper care after heart attack, between 3 to 12 months, can reduce the risk of MI.
16. Adults living in less walkable neighborhoods had a higher risk of heart failure.
17. Low-load blood flow restricted resistance exercise (BFRRE) can increase the quality of a life for heart patients.
18. Hormone replacement therapy increases the risk of MI.
19. Illicit drug use.
20. A history of preeclampsia.
21. An autoimmune condition.
22. Patients with advanced chronic kidney disease sustain extremely high mortality rates following acute myocardial infarction.
23. Stress.
24. MI occurring between 6 am and noon are associated with the most damage.
25. Link between abdominal fat and repeat heart attacks.
26. Heart attack without having blocked arteries. Is this possible?
27. Diabetes independently linked to increased heart failure.
28. Generic blood pressure drugs remain in a big problem.
29. Fatigue/heartburn/discomfort in chest, back and jaw/shortness of breath (Silent MI).
30. Deficiency in Vitamin D3.
31. Eating eggs might not be so bad for you, but they still affect cholesterol.
32. Aspirin does not always help the heart and may hurt by causing increased bleeding.

33. Fish oil is helpful if you have coronary artery disease and high triglycerides.
34. Take your blood pressure medications at night.
35. Drug may compromise cardiovascular health.
36. High blood pressure.
37. ECG.
38. Blood tests for heart disease.
    - Total cholesterol.
    - Low-density lipoprotein (LDL) cholesterol.
    - High-density lipoprotein (HDL).
    - Triglycerides.
    - Non-HDL cholesterol.
39. High-sensitivity C-reactive protein.
    - A hs-CRP level.
    - Lipoprotein.
    - Plasma ceramides.
    - Natriuretic peptides.
    - Troponin T.

It is important to convert these statistics into knowledge, which is possible only with the help of expertise in this domain. A survey form is circulated to the experts for the same. Though many parameters are responsible for MI, a few of much importance were concluded from the assessment.

Step B: Survey on Expertise Inputs

Figures 7.10 and 7.11 (a–h) show the most preferred and plausible parameter for detection of MI by professionals, ECG being the most logical one and cholesterol the least. However, all the parameters are given equal importance

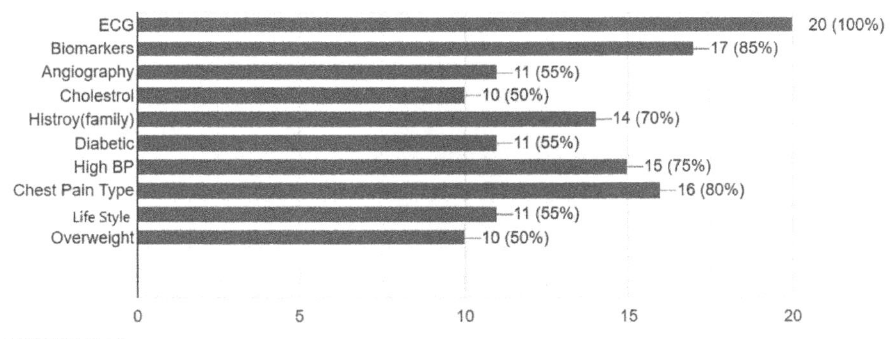

FIGURE 7.10
Bar Graph for MI Parameters.

Link between abdominal fat and repeat heart attacks.

22 responses

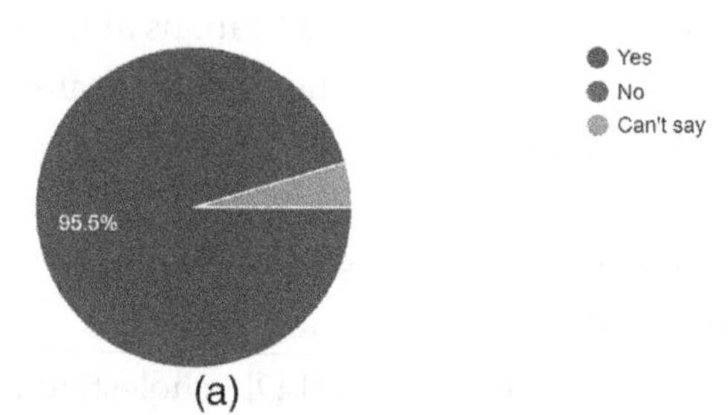

(a)

Fatigue/heartburn/discomfort in chest, back and jaw/shortness of breath (Silent MI)

22 responses

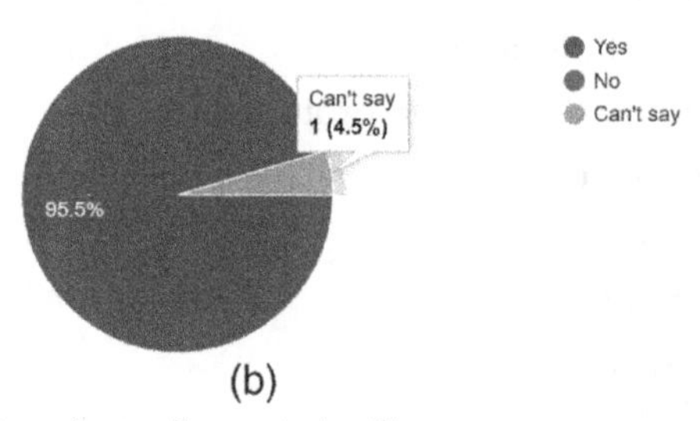

(b)

Drugs may compromise cardiovascular health

22 responses

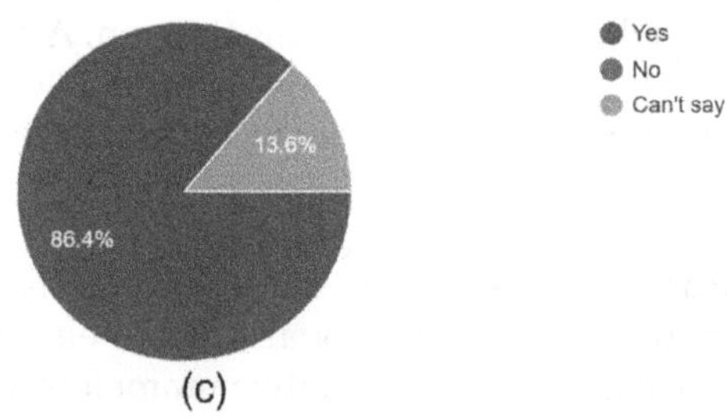

(c)

In heart failure (HF), cardiac energy metabolism is deranged

22 responses

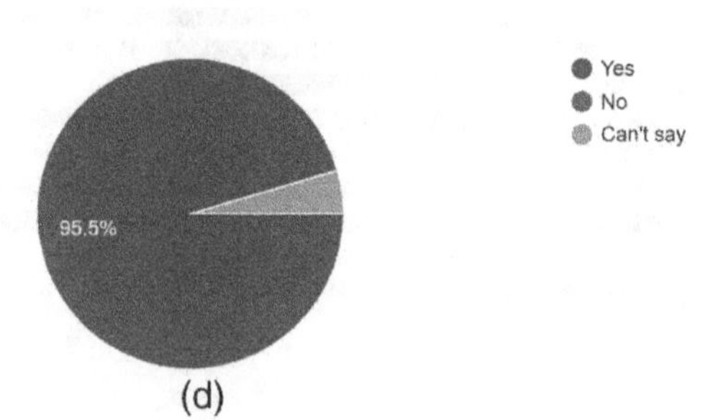

(d)

FIGURE 7.11 (A–H)
Survey Pie Charts.

Heart attack without having blocked arteries. Is this possible?

22 responses

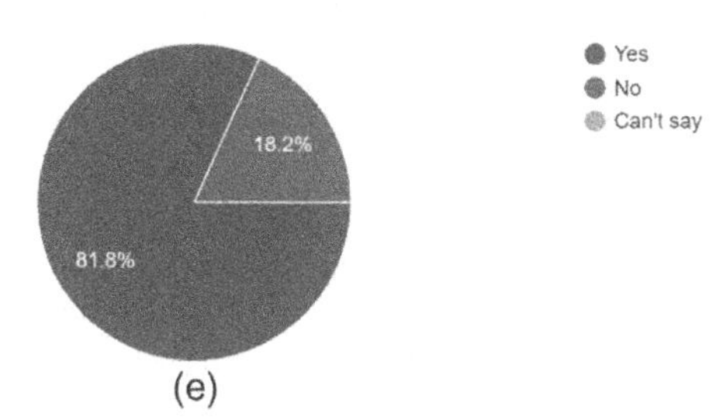

Proper care after heart attack between 3 to 12 months can reduce the risk of MI

22 responses

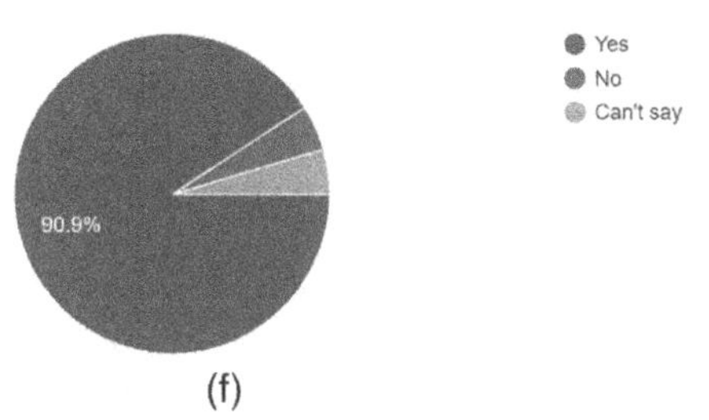

Thyroid dysfunction

22 responses

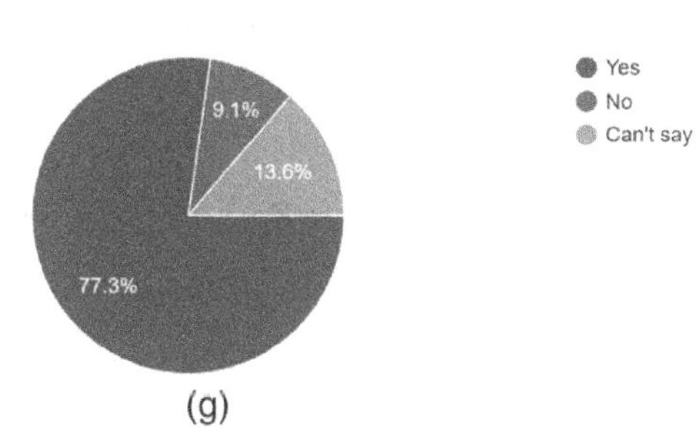

HF is associated with increased risk of maternal mortality and morbidities

22 responses

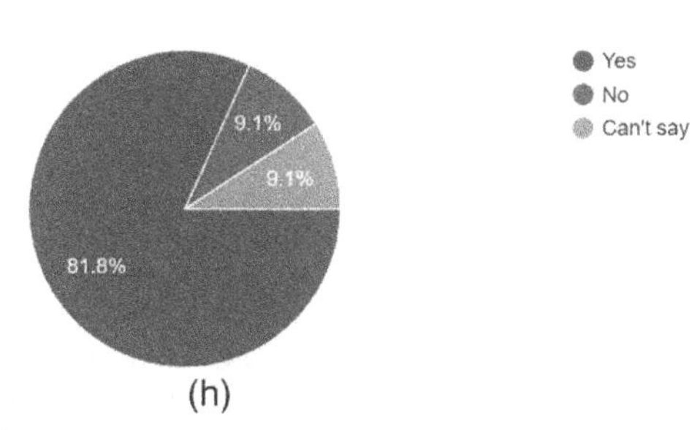

FIGURE 7.11 (A–H) (Continued)
Survey Pie Charts.

in this research for more accuracy. Parameters contributing significantly in the detection of MI are excerpted and describe here.

Pie chart above shows the relation of chronic kidney disease and acute myocardial infarction as observed in patients according to the professionals that had filled the survey form; 94.7 percent of them agreed to the relation between the two diseases.

One of the pie charts depicts that patients undergoing stress are more prone to heart diseases, according to our professionals and their experiences; 94.7 percent of experts believe that patients having abdominal fat and are overweight are prone to repeated heart attacks. However, a few of them aren't sure about the relation between the two.

Various drugs available today for different diseases have their own side effects, one of them being a compromise on cardiovascular health. The same is shown in the above chart.

Diverse surgeries and procedures have their own disadvantages, which might become a cause of further heart failure in the near future of the patient; 73.7 percent of experts believe this to be true, however a few disapprove the same and the rest aren't sure.

All the metabolism and functions in our body are related to one another directly or indirectly. Dysfunction of one may be the cause of failure of the other. Similarly, there might be a relation between thyroid dysfunction and heart diseases as observed from the pie chart above.

Most illicit drugs are not considered good for the body, and so it is obvious for them to have a negative effect on a vital organ like the heart. However only 50 percent professionals think this to be true while the rest are unsure about it.

Step C: Excerption of Parameters Based on Above Survey

1. Age.
2. Sex.
3. ECG.
4. Biomarkers (CK-MB, TROP-I).
5. Angiography (LAD, LCA, RCA).
6. Cholesterol.
7. Bp (Systolic, Diastolic).
8. Chest pain type (Acute, Chronic).
9. Diabetic (Yes, No).
10. History: Chronic kidney disease, autoimmune condition, previous heart failure (PHF), ischemic heart disease (IHD), hormone replacement therapy, thyroid dysfunction, acute kidney injury.

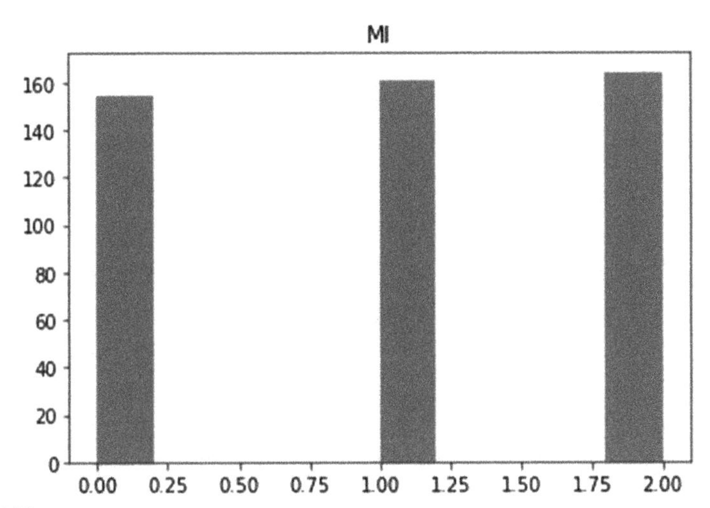

FIGURE 7.12
Balanced Dataset.

11. MI or early MI (Early MI=0, MI=1).

Step D: Data Gathering
Raw data is collected from various hospitals. This data is available in the form of images as shown in Figure 7.13.

Step E: Data Reading
The data available in the form of images was read and transfigured into an Excel file with the aid of expertise as shown in Figure 7.14.

Step F: Data Normalization and Bucketization
The data is shown in Figure 7.15.

7.6.2 Experimental Result

The data assembled from hospitals are used to train the model, and Table 7.4 shows its accuracy while training and testing. However, this table is giving 100 percent accuracy due to overfitting, the main cause of which is a smaller count of samples provided to the proposed model. Accuracy of the model is directly proportional to the data and samples fed to it. This gives us a future scope of improved accuracy as a result of relevant data given. In spite of using actual dataset of patients from the hospital of recent years (2019–2020), and constant support and feedback from the expertise, the model is not accurate due to overfitting. This can be overcome by increasing the number of sample dataset entered in the model in the near future. It is also necessary to apply other models such as ensemble algorithm and neural network to get the best accuracy.

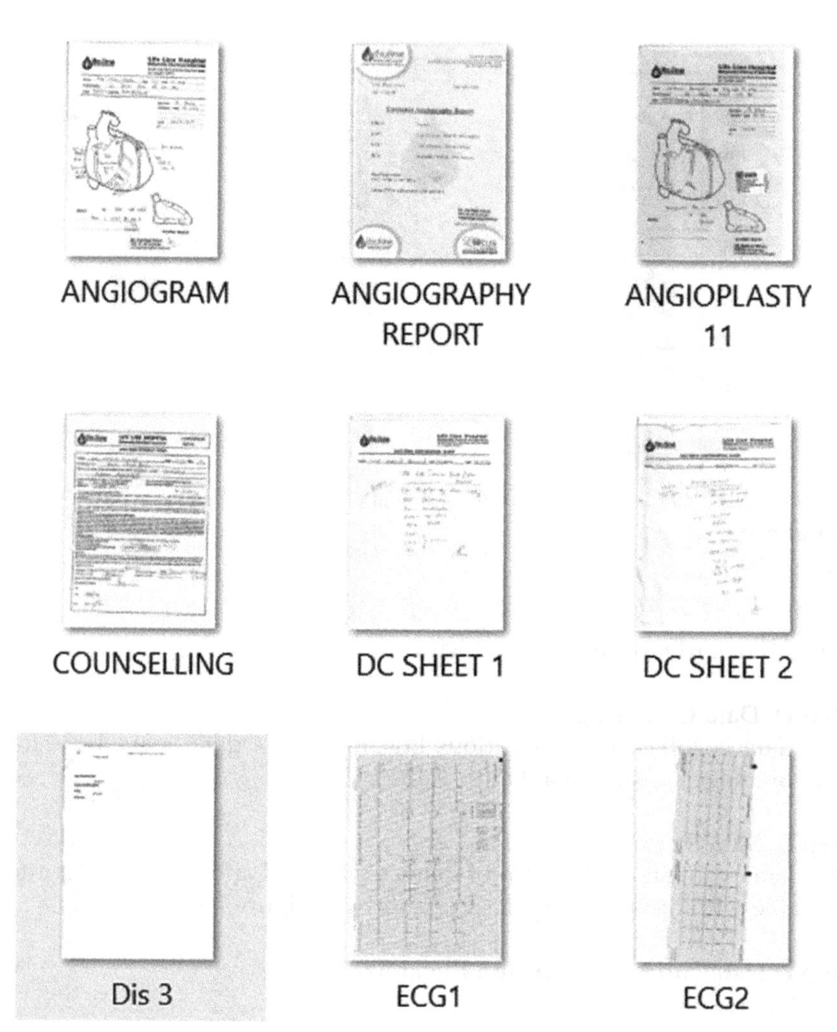

FIGURE 7.13
Patients Report.

age	sex	ecg changes	biomarkers		angiography			bp		chestpai	diabetic	Chol	CKD	AC	PHForIHD	Hor_Rep	Thy_dys	AKI	mi
			CK-MB	TROP-I	LAD	LCA	RCA	SYS	DIAS										
49	1	1	0	0	0.35	0.25	0	125	75	2	1	180	0	0	0	1	0	0	0
57	1	0	0	0	0.9	0	0.2	130	70	2	0	195	0	0	0	0	0	1	0
49	1	1	0	0	0.5	0	0	130	80	2	1	210	0	0	0	0	0	1	0
47	0	1	1	1	0.7	0	0.8	135	85	2	1	190	0	0	0	0	1	0	0
45	1	0	1	1	0.5	0.3	0	145	90	2	1	223	0	0	0	0	0	0	0
57	1	1	1	0	0.9	0	0	120	80	2	0	175	0	0	1	0	0	1	1
60	1	1	0	0	0.65	0.99	0	130	90	2	0	280	0	0	1	0	0	0	1
70	1	1	1	1	0.85	0	0	140	90	2	0	230	0	0	0	0	0	1	1
56	0	1	0	0	0	0.9	1	130	90	2	1	222	0	1	0	0	1	0	1
49	1	1	0	0	0	0	1	130	80	2	0	243	0	0	1	0	0	0	1
50	1	1	0	0	0.85	0.85	0	140	90	2	0	267	0	0	0	0	0	1	1
60	1	1	1	1	0	0	0.8	140	90	2	1	250	0	0	0	0	0	1	1

FIGURE 7.14
Patients Report into Excel.

age	sex	ecg chang	CK-MB	TROP-I	LAD	LCA	RCA	SYS	DIAS	chestpain	diabetic	Chol	CKD	AC	PHForIHD	Hor_Rep	Thy_dys	AKI	mi
63	1	1	1	1	0.9	0	0.9	220	120	1	0	231	1	0	1	0	0	0	1
54	1	1	1	1	0.9	0	1	140	90	2	1	250	0	0	0	0	0	1	1
49	1	1	0	0	0.8	0.5	0	160	90	2	0	195	0	1	0	1	0	0	0
48	1	1	0	0	0.8	0.5	0	140	100	2	0	195	0	1	0	1	0	0	0
52	0	0	0	0	0	0.3	0	170	90	2	1	200	0	0	0	0	1	0	0
45	0	0	0	0	0.7	0.3	0	150	100	2	1	200	0	0	0	0	1	0	0
72	1	1	1	1	0	0	0.9	150	90	1	0	190	0	0	0	0	0	0	1
63	1	1	1	1	0.85	0	0	160	90	2	1	209	1	0	1	0	0	1	1
50	1	1	1	1	0.9	0.7	0	170	90	1	0	190	0	1	0	0	0	0	1
55	1	1	0	0	0	0.2	0.5	150	100	2	1	150	0	0	0	1	0	0	0
54	1	1	0	0	0	0.2	0.5	160	90	2	1	150	0	0	0	1	0	0	0
58	0	0	0	0	0.4	0.2	0	160	100	2	0	200	0	1	0	0	0	0	0
41	0	0	0	0	0.4	0.2	0	170	90	2	0	200	0	1	0	0	0	0	0

FIGURE 7.15
Patients Report into Excel.

TABLE 7.4

Comparison of Algorithms

Algorithms	Training Set (%)	Testing Set (%)
SVM	58.62	62.52
NAÏVE BAYES	100.0	75.0
LOGISTIC REGRESSION	100.0	87.5
DECISION TREE	100.0	87.5
RANDOM FOREST	100.0	87.5

TABLE 7.5

Comparison of Algorithms [Enhanced Result]

Algorithms	Training Set (%)	Testing Set (%)
SVM	67.33	63.00
NAÏVE BAYES	48.99	47.00
LOGISTIC REGRESSION	65.07	62.00
DECISION TREE	67.58	62.00
RANDOM FOREST	67.58	63.00

7.6.3 Enhanced Experimental Result

Table 7.5 shows the accuracy better than Table 7.4. This is achieved by increasing the number of samples fed to the model along with the continuous support and feedback of expertise. This clearly shows that overfitting can be removed by increasing the number of inputs given to the model.

It is also necessary to apply other models such as ensemble algorithm and neural network to get better accuracy.

7.7 Conclusion and Future Scope

In this research on detection of myocardial infarction, the existing dataset of only four places were taken into consideration based on their availability. Due to this restriction, the datasets of all the four were merged giving us a less accurate result due to overfitting of the model. This hinders the process of diagnosis and cannot be relied upon. To overcome this problem of overfitting of the model, transferring this information into a graph showed that Cleveland had the least number of missing values. As a result, all the machine learning algorithms – such as SVM, Naïve Bayes, Decision Tree, Random Forest and Logistic Regression – were applied only on dataset of the Cleveland. On application of the same, SVM gave the most accurate results.

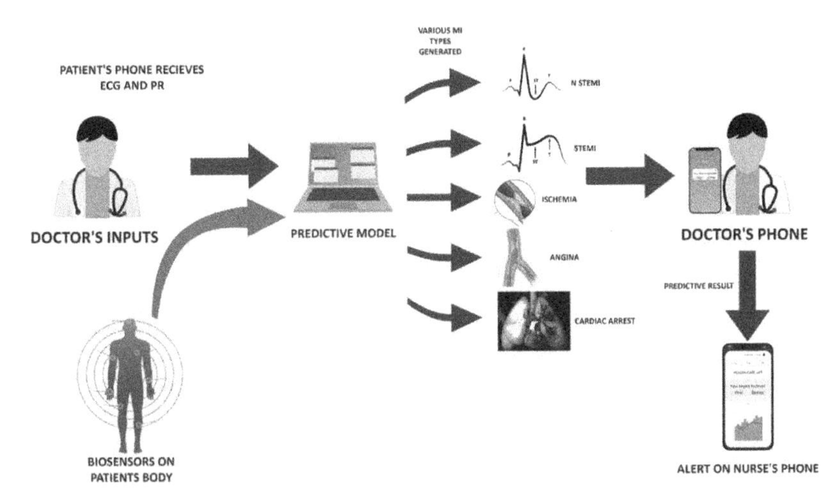

FIGURE 7.16
Schematic Diagram.

Constant discussion with the experts and consideration of new reports for early detection of MI, gave us new parameters to be added in this dataset with reference to India. After cleaning and pruning of raw data received in the form of images, that data was fed to the model for application of algorithms, the results of which was not as accurate as expected due to overfitting. The only reason for this issue is a smaller number of samples given to the model, which can be overcome by adding more datasets and feedback from the doctor. Also, other classifiers have to apply to increase the accuracy. Ensemble algorithm and neural network are suggested to use in further research work.

7.7.1 Future Scope

Throwing light on the future scope of this model, on successful application and receiving accurate data as expected, the model can directly read the data required from the patient's body for detection of (early) MI and provide us with immediate results for the necessary actions needed to be taken by the patient or the hospital staff in any unforeseen situation. The model will provide an easy way for the patients to keep a check on their heart disease and monitor if they have MI, at their own convenience. (Refer to Figure 7.16)

References

[1] Westwood, James D., Helene M. Hoffman, Richard A. Robb, & Don Stredeny *Medicine Meets Virtual Reality, Applying Moore's Law to Health*. 1999, IOS Press.

[2] Bonow, Mann, & Libby Zipes, "Heart Disease," *A Textbook of Cardiovascular Medicine*, 9th Edition, 2011.

[3] www.youtube.com/watch?v=2kLlhlsesRQ.

[4] Groennebaek, Thomas, Peter Sieljacks, Roni Nielsen, Kasper Pryds, Nichlas R. Jespersen, Jakob Wang, Caroline R. Carlsen, Michael R. Schmidt, Frank V. de Paoli, Benjamin F. Miller, Kristian Vissing, & Hans Erik Bøtker, "Effect of Blood Flow Restricted Resistance Exercise and Remote Ischemic Conditioning on Functional Capacity and Myocellular Adaptations in Patients with Heart Failure," *Circulation: Heart Failure* 2019; 12: e 006427. DOI: 10.1161/CIRCHEARTFAILURE.119.006427 December 2019.

[5] Howell, Nicholas A., Jack V. Tu, Rahim Moineddin, Anna Chu, & Gillian L. Booth, "Association Between Neighborhood Walkability and Predicted 10-Year Cardiovascular Disease Risk: The CANHEART (Cardiovascular Health in Ambulatory Care Research Team) Cohort," *Journal of the American Heart Association*, December 2019.

[6] Liu, Junfeng, Lukai Zheng, Yajun Cheng, Shuting Zhang, Bo Wu, Deren Wang, Shihong Zhang, Wendan Tao, Simiao Wu, & Ming Liu, "Trends in Outcomes of Patients With Ischemic Stroke Treated Between 2002 and 2016," *Circulation: Heart Failure.* 2019; 12: e005610. DOI:10.1161/CIRCOUTCOMES.119.005610 December 2019.

[7] Bertero, Edoardo, Vasco Sequeira, & Christoph Maack, "Hungry Hearts," *Circulation: Heart Failure.* 2018; 11: e005642. DOI: 10.1161/CIRCHEARTFAILURE.118.005642 December 2018.

[8] Kannan, Lakshmi, Pamela A. Shaw, Michael P. Morley, Jeffrey Brandimarto, James C. Fang, Nancy K. Sweitzer, Thomas P. Cappola, & Anne R. Cappola, "Thyroid Dysfunction in Heart Failure and Cardiovascular Outcomes," *Circulation: Heart Failure.* 2018; 11: e005266.DOI:10.1161/CIRCHEARTFAILURE.118.005266 December 2018.

[9] Mogos, Mulubrhan F., Mariann R. Piano, Barbara L. McFarlin, Jason L. Salemi, Kylea L. Liese, & Joan E. Briller, "Heart Failure in Pregnant Women A Concern Across the Pregnancy Continuum," *Circulation: Heart Failure.* 2018; 11: e004005. DOI: 10.1161/CIRCHEARTFAILURE.117.004005, January 2018.

[10] Thorvaldsen, Tonje, Brian L. Claggett, Amil Shah, Susan Cheng, Sunil K. Agarwal, Lisa M. Wruck, Patricia P. Chang, Wayne D. Rosamond, Eldrin F. Lewis, Akshay S. Desai, Lars H. Lund, & Scott D. Solomon, "Predicting Risk in Patients Hospitalized for Acute Decompensated Heart Failure and Preserved Ejection Fraction," *Circulation: Heart Failure.* 2017; 10: e003992. DOI: 10.1161/CIRCHEARTFAILURE.117.003992 December 2017.

[11] Egbe, Alexander C., Heidi M. Connolly, William R. Miranda, Naser M. Ammash, Donald J. Hagler, Gruschen R. Veldtman, & Barry A. Borlaug, "Hemo dynamics of Fontan Failure the Role of Pulmonary Vascular Disease," *Circulation: Heart Failure.* 2017; 10: e004515. DOI: 10.1161/CIRCHEARTFAILURE.117. 004515, December 2017.

[12] Uchihashi, Motoki, Atsushi Hoshino, Yoshifumi Okawa, Makoto Ariyoshi, Satoshi Kaimoto, Shuhei Tateishi, Kazunori Ono, Ryoetsu Yamanaka, Daichi Hato, Yohei Fushimura, Sakiko Honda, Kuniyoshi Fukai, Yusuke Higuchi, Takehiro Ogata, Eri Iwai-Kanai, & Satoaki Matoba, "Cardiac-Specific Bdh1 Overexpression Ameliorates Oxidative Stress and Cardiac Remodeling

in Pressure Overload–Induced Heart Failure," *Circulation: Heart Failure.* 2017; 10: e004417. DOI: 10.1161/CIRCHEARTFAILURE.117.004417, December 2017.

[13] Jessup, Mariell, & Elliott Antman, *Reducing the Risk of Heart Attack and Stroke – The American Heart Association/American College of Cardiology Prevention Guidelines.* 2014, American Heart Association.

[14] Williams, Redford B. *Depression After Heart Attack – Why Should I Be Concerned about Depression After a Heart Attack?* 2011, American Heart Association.

[15] Chaturvedi, Seemant. *Should Stroke Be Considered Both a Brain Attack and a Heart Attack?* 2007, American Heart Association.

[16] Stern, Michael D. *How to Give a Cell a Heart Attack.* 2006, American Heart Association.

[17] Becker, Richard C. *Heart Attack and Stroke Prevention in Women.* 2005, American Heart Association.

[18] Ornato, Joseph P. & Mary M. Hand, *Warning Signs of a Heart Attack.* 2001 American Heart Association.

[19] Khaw, Kay-Tee & Elizabeth Barrett-Connor, "Family History of Heart Attack: A Modifiable Risk Factor?" *Journals of the American Heart Association* 74(2), August 1986.

[20] Barrett-Connor, Elizabeth & Kay-Tee Khaw, "Family History of Heart Attack as an Independent Predictor of Death Due to Cardiovascular Disease," *Journals of the American Heart Association* 69(6), 1984.

[21] www.webmd.com/sex-relationships/features/mimi-guarneri#3

[22] Charrad, Tesnim, Kaouther Nouira, & Ahmed Ferchichi, "Use of Hierarchical Temporal Memory Algorithm in Heart Attack Detection," *World Academy of Science, Engineering and Technology International Journal of Computer and Systems Engineering* 13(5), 2019.

[23] Singh, Reetu & E. Rajesh, "Prediction of Heart Disease by Clustering and Classification Techniques," *International Journal of Computer Sciences and Engineering* 7(5), 2019.

[24] Kumar, Vikas, Praveen Kumar, & Masoud Mohammadian, "Formulation of an Elegant Diagnostic Approach for an Intelligent Disease Recommendation System," 2019, 9th international Conference IEEE.

[25] Faus, Oliver, Yuki Hagiwara, Tan Jen Hong, Oh Shu Lih,& U Rajendra Acharya, "Deep Learning for Healthcare applications Based on Physiological Signals", *Computer Methods and Programs in Biomedicine,* 161, 2018: 1–13.

[26] Raju, Cincy, Philipsy E., Siji Chacko, L. Padma Suresh, Deepa Rajan S., "A Survey on Predicting Heart Disease using Data Mining Techniques, Proc. IEEE Conference on Emerging Devices and Smart Systems ICEDSS 2018.

[27] Jabbar, M.A., B.L Deek Shatulu, & Priti Chndra, "Alternating Decision Trees for Early Diagnosis of Heart Disease," Proceedings of International Conference on Circuits, Communication, Control and Computing, 2014.

[28] Shehnai, Bandarage & Gamage Upeksha Ganegoda, "Heart Diseases Prediction with Data Mining and Neural Network Techniques," 3rd International Conference for Convergence in Technology (I2CT), 2018.

[29] Revathi, J. & J. Anitha, "A Survey on Analysis of ST-Segment to Diagnose Coronary Artery Disease," International Conference on Signal Processing and Communication (ICSPC'17) – 28 & 29 July 2017.

[30] Tikotikar, Ahelam & Mallikarjun Kodabagi, "A Survey on Technique for Prediction of Disease in Medical Data," 2017 International Conference on Smart Technologies for Smart Nation.

[31] Gowrishankar S., Prachita M.Y., & Arvind Prakash, "IoT based Heart Attack Detection, Heart Rate and Temperature Monitor," *International Journal of Computer Applications* 170(5), July 2017.

[32] Hazra, Animesh, Subrata Kumar Mandal, Amit Gupta, Arkomita Mukherjee, & Asmita Mukherjee "Heart Disease Diagnosis and Prediction Using Machine Learning and Data Mining Techniques: A Review," 10(7) 2017.

[33] Anbarasi, A. & Ravi Subban, "Abnormalities in Mitral Valve of Heart Detection and Analysis using Echocardiography Images," 2017 IEEE International Conference on Computational Intelligence and Computing Research (ICCIC).

[34] Bisen, Priti & Mahesh Pawar, "Monitoring and Recording of Critical Parameters of Human Using KY202," International Conference on Innovations in Information, Embedded and Communication Systems (ICIIECS), 2017.

[35] Gnaneswar, B., & M.R. Ebenezar Jebarani, "A Review on Prediction and Diagnosis of Heart Failure," International Conference on Innovations in Information, Embedded and Communication System (ICIIECS), 2017.

[36] Sharma, Richa, Shailendra Narayan Singh, & Sujata Khatri, "Medical Data Mining Using Different Classification and Clustering Techniques: A Critical Survey," Second International Conference on Computational Intelligence & Communication Technology, 2016.

[37] Singh, Manpreet, Levi Monteiro Martins, Patrick Joanis & Vijay K. Mago "Building a Cardiovascular Disease Predictive Model using Structural Equation Model & Fuzzy Cognitive Map," 2016 IEEE International Conference on Fuzzy Systems (FUZZ-IEEE).

[38] Ahmed, Wakas & Shezad Khalid, "ECG Signal Processing for Recognition of Cardiovascular Diseases: A Survey," The Sixth International Conference on Innovative Computing Technology INTECH, 2016.

[39] Salma Banu, N.K., & Suma Swamy, "Prediction of Heart Disease at early stage using Data Mining and Big Data Analytics: A Survey," International Conference on Electrical, Electronics, Communication, Computer and Optimization Techniques (ICEECCOT), 2016.

[40] Haritha, C., & M. Ganesan, "A Survey on Modern Trends in ECG Noise Removal Techniques." International Conference on Circuit, Power and Computing Technologies (ICCPCT) 2016.

[41] Bonaca, Marc P., J. Antonio Gutierrez, Mark A. Creager, Benjamin M. Scirica, Jeffrey Olin, Sabina A. Murphy, Eugene Braunwald, & David A. Morrow, "Acute Limb Ischemia and Outcomes with Vorapaxar in Patients with Peripheral Artery Disease," American Heart Association, 2016.

[42] Princy, R. Theresa & J. Thomas, "Human Heart Disease Prediction System Using Data Mining Techniques," International Conference on Circuit, Power and Computing Technologies (ICCPCT) 2016.

[43] Duchateau, Nicolas, Mathieu De Craene, Pascal Allain, Eric Saloux, & Maxime Sermesant "Infarct Localization from Myocardial Deformation," IEEE Transactions on Medical Imaging, 2016.

[44] Silverberg, J. I. "Association between Adult Atopic Dermatitis, Cardiovascular Disease, and Increased Heart Attacks in Three Population-based Studies," *Allergy* 70: 1300–1308, 2015, John Wiley.

[45] Jambukia, Shweta H. Vipul K. Dhabi, & Harshadkumar B. Prajapati, "Classification of ECG signals using Machine Learning Techniques: A Survey," International Conference on Advances in Computer Engineering and Applications (ICACEA) 2015.

[46] www.google.co.in/search?q=feature+selection+in+machine+learning&dcr=0&sxsrf=ALeKk01e9wpV-V0YyXnAtW_4uYn1de_eoA:1599282930163&source=lnms&tbm=isch&sa=X&ved=2ahUKEwiRh8qXodHrAhV5zjgGHT4LCTwQ_AUoAXoECBAQAw&biw=1280&bih=578

8

Diagnostics and Decision Support for Cardiovascular System: A Tool Based on PPG Signature

Palash Kumar Kundu and Madhusree Kundu

CONTENTS

8.1 Introduction and Background

The semantic origin of photoplethysmography (PPG) has a lineage to the combination of *photo*, meaning light; *plethysmo*, meaning blood; and *graphy*, meaning measurement. Over the last few decades, cardiovascular diseases (CVDs) have emerged as one of the most fatal ailments all over the world. The deaths of nearly 23.6 million people by the year 2030 due to cardiovascular ailments are predicted. South-East Asia may be the epicenter of these diseases [1].

Continuous health-care monitoring can reduce the risk factors behind CVDs. Continual health-care monitoring in remote locations, especially people in rural areas of developing countries, is a staggering task due to high population density, lack of proper health-care policies and infrastructural facilities, and to an inadequate number of medical practitioners [2]. Under such circumstances, interactive patient-care tools developed using various biomedical signals, including PPG signals, may to a certain degree help local medical practitioners in supplementing their medical judgment.

Biomedical signals are observations of physiological activities of organisms, which include gene and protein expressions, neural and cardiac leaps, and images of organs and tissues. With the Internet of things available, treatment also can be conducted from any distant, convenient and urban locations consulting the concerned experienced physicians. It is appropriate here to mention that biomedical signals (physical and behavioral features) may be deployed as an identity detector. PPG may serve as a unique biometric identifier for individuals deciphering various phases of this waveform.

There has been an increasing demand for an innovative, non-invasive, inexpensive and rapid-method / device targeting automated diagnosis and decision support in treating cardiovascular ailments [3]. Clinical inferences on cardiac health have been depending on electrocardiograph (ECG) for quite some time now. Due to the effect of noise, motion artefact and diverse morphological characteristic of ECG waveform, an alternate, easy-to-implementation bio-waveform based techniques such as PPG has been elicited in the diagnosis and prognosis of cardiac ailments. Due to the discomfort of cuff-based blood pressure measurement, PPG based measurement of blood pressure is emerging [4].

Hardware requirements of PPG signal generation is comparatively simpler than ECG, and the proposed device is a wearable one. The photoplethysmogram was captured using an infrared light source (through a photodiode releasing 900 nm wavelength light) and a detector (phototransistor). PPG waveform measurements are of two types: transmission (PPGT, where detection is done by placing source and detector in parallel to each other) and reflection (PPGR, where source and detector are flanked side by side).

PPG rhythm is generated by heart muscle contraction directing blood flow to the fringe tissues. Blood movement through arteries resembles pulsatile flow, hence reflectance and transmittance of light emitted by arteries depends on the volume of blood passing through them at that moment [1]. The high-frequency (HF) AC segment of the PPG signal designates absorbance due to blood flow through the artery, and a low-frequency (LF) AC signal originates from blood flow through veins and the DC component of it (describing the fixed quantity of blood flowing through the artery and other constant tissue optical factors, including skin pigmentation and hemoglobin) [5]. The AC segment of the PPG signal is the provider of characteristic fiducial points pertaining to the systolic and diastolic components [6–7]. Apart from that, PPG signal consists of noise caused by poor perfusion rate and motion artefact [8].

PPG signatures may be collected from ear lobe or fingertip. Aortic notch or dicrotic notch (resembles the arterial elasticity) are minor ricochets that separate the arterial pulse into systolic and diastolic phases (Figure 8.1). The first and second order derivatives of PPG waveform provide better fiducial features. Second order derivative of PPG (SDPPG), or acceleration PPG, is analyzed using the amplitudes of distinct waves – namely, "wave a" (premature positive systolic wave), "wave b" (initial negative systolic wave), "wave c" (mature re-soaring systolic wave), "wave d" (mature re-decreasing systolic wave) and "wave e" (premature diastolic positive wave), representing the dicrotic notch [9]. All b, c, d, and e waves are normalized, by dividing them by a. The characteristic amplitudes *A*b and *A*d are normalized b and d waves, named as *PPG Ab* and *PPG Ad*, respectively. PPGAI index is derived as:

$$PPGAI = \frac{PPG\,Ad}{PPG\,Ab}$$

PPGAI index is calculated for each waveform from the PPG signal and the results are averaged with the standard deviation being estimated. PPGAI is one of the significant monitoring parameters for premature arterial stiffness, hence, suspected cardiovascular aging. The standard deviations were calculated for the *PPGAI* of each subject. Instant heart rate is derived as (60/PP), where PP is the interval between beats is and expressed in seconds. The pulse-to-pulse interval (PP) is derived from the PPG signal, which is sensitive to breathing-interval changes and a useful indicator for the variation/non-linearity of pulse rate. Figure 8.1 represents fiducial points of interest from 1st and 2nd derivative of PPG signal from a 57-year-old volunteer.

Heart-rate variability (HRV) refers to the deviations in time interludes between successive heartbeats. A healthy heart manifests non-linear, oscillating characteristics. This non-linear rhythm of the heart allows the cardiovascular system to ratify any abrupt challenges [10]. Heart-rate variability (HRV) is a widespread non-invasive indicator used to review cardiac health. The autonomic nervous system ensures coordination between the central nervous system and the cardiovascular system [1]. HRV using PPG signals can be measured either by (a) extents of the PP intervals or the instant heart rate (60/PP), and by (b) the alterations between PP intermissions.

In 1965 Hon and Lee [11] evaluated the clinical significance of HRV for the first time and observed alterations in inter-beat intervals before fatal cardiac arrest without any palpable change in the heart rate itself. Only after 1980 was the clinical significance of HRV established when a strong correlation was established between HRV and mortality following an acute myocardial infarction [12–14].

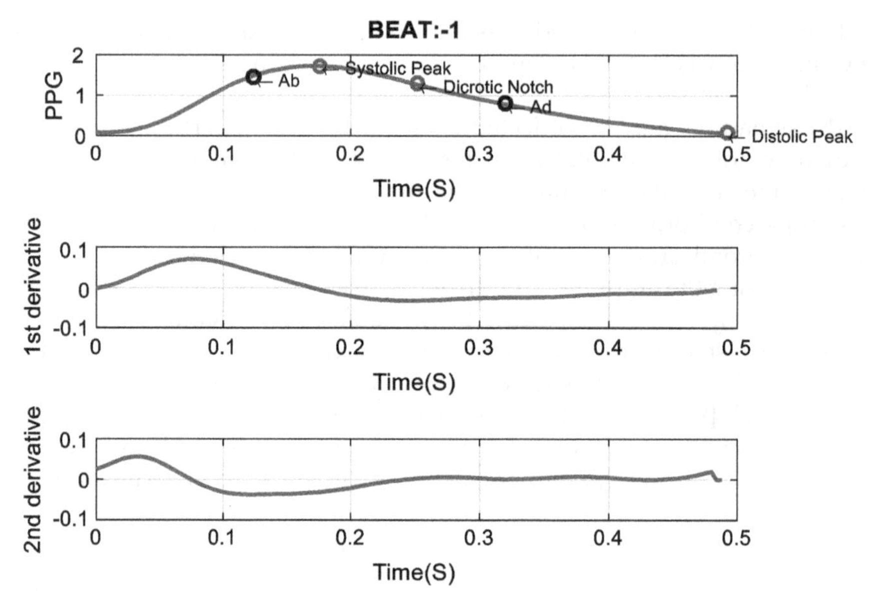

FIGURE 8.1
Fiducial Points from BEAT 1 of PPG Signal of 57-year-old Subject.

HRV derived from ECG is the time lag fringed between successive R waves. The non-linearity present in the inter-beat striding intervals of heart oscillations are clinically relevant for investigative and predictive purposes. Recently. PPG (in terms of peak-to-peak interval signals) has been projected as a substitute for ECG in HRV measurement [15]. It may be pertinent to mention that depolarization and repolarization of the heart instigates the spread of the pulsatile wave of blood to the edges. This pulse propagation time owes for a minor (a few milliseconds) difference [16–18] in heartbeat intermissions derived from ECG and PPG. Such small variations between the two approaches may not be appreciable in the time-domain analysis, but be prominent in non-linear HRV analysis and its interpretation in the frequency domain. Therein lies connectivity between ECG and PPG through formidable correspondence between the RR intermissions (ECG-derived) and PP intermissions (PPG-derived). PP variability was precise (0.1 ms) as compared to RR variability. HRV parameters estimated in time and frequency domain using RR and PP interval methods revealed no significant differences ($p < 0.05$) [17].

The time domain, HRV metrics, consists of SDPP (Standard deviation of PP intermissions), pPP50 (fraction of consecutive PP intermissions that differ by more than 50 ms out of all PP intermissions), RMSSD (Root mean square of successive PP interval differences) and so forth, parameters. Time-domain indices monitoring periods ranging from ~2 min to 24 h.

Two coinciding processes of distinct origin are responsible for ECG-based short-range HRV measurements. One of the processes is owing to interaction between sympathetic and parasympathetic nervous systems. The other process refers to the regulatory mechanisms controlling heart rate via various mechanisms related to the cardiac cycle [10]. The 24 h HRV recording is regarded as the "golden routine" for determining heart rate variability [10].

Frequency-domain measurements estimate the total HRV power spanned over four frequency bands (ms^2/Hz), namely, ultra-low-frequency (ULF), very-low-frequency (VLF), low-frequency (LF), and high-frequency (HF) bands [19]. For short-range HRV measurements, frequency–domain methods are preferred [10]. Capturing span for HRV frequency-band measurements are documented [10].

Jermana L. Moraes et al. [1] presented a review of the PPG technique including a comparative study with the ECG technique, and most important variables that may be harnessed using the PPG signal.

PPG technology is an easy-to-implement and cost-effective technology that can be harnessed for cardiac health monitoring (oxygen saturation level of blood, heart rate, blood pressure (BP), arterial stiffening due to age etc.) [20]. PPG and ECG jointly may monitor cardiac arrhythmia. PPG can be deployed to assess the ventilator-driven inflections associated with hypovolemia [21].

In addition to clinical situations, sports persons, exercise enthusiasts and elderly individuals need real-time conditions for their HR to avoid risky physical activity, hence, avoiding chances of a fatal heart attack. PPG signals monitor with precision HR in rest positions, adapting them in dynamic situations; but this monitoring remains challenging because of motion artefacts (MA) corrupting the signals (Khan et al., 2015) [22–23].

The Poincaré plot states the relationship between consecutive sample points in time-series data. Physiological rhythms exhibit auto-correlation behavior depicting a memory process. The Poincaré plot already had been harnessed in clinical investigations due to bodily fluctuations [24]. Short- and long-range variability in any physical rhythm revealed as a Poincaré plot is defined as standard deviations perpendicular and parallel to the line of identity [25]. The Poincaré plot has the ability to establish correlation behavior among discrete signal values in a time-series (Pearson's correlation coefficient, r). Satti et al. (2019) presented Poincaré method applications for heart-rate variability in patients with various chronic diseases [26]. For asthmatics, an extended Poincaré plot was used as a non-invasive means to classify among respiratory diseases [26].

In this very perspective, a PPG waveform-based cardiovascular diagnostic tool has been developed consisting of several modules. The present chapter on indigenous PPG waveform-based automated cardiovascular diagnostic tool is being framed as follows: Section 8.2 presents the PPG data acquisition system; Section 8.3 describes data pre-processing/conditioning; and PPG beat extraction is addressed in Section 8.4. Section 8.5 analyses the extracted PPG waveforms and estimates clinical parameters using the fiducial points of PPG and its second-order derivative, SDPPG. HRV estimations in time and non-linear domain including Poincaŕe plots are described in Section 8.6. In an ending note, Section 8.7 summarizes the results, accompanied by discussion; the chapter concludes with Section 8.8. All the algorithms involved in various sections were implemented on a MATLAB environment leading to an automated system.

8.2 PPG Data Acquisition System

PPG waveforms were recorded from the fingertips of 15 subjects in pertinent age groups: 11–12 years, 21–25 years, 35–40 years and 50–62 years. A reflectance and finger type PPG sensor unit including IR transmitter and receiver placed at their proximity was deployed. The amount of light transmitted across the finger was subjected to the blood-volume pertaining in the tissue. The output of the sensor was connected to an analog channel of a TMEGA328 (ARDUINO UNO R3) embedded controller (Figure 8.2). A data-capture program written in embedded C (ARDUINO C) was used to collect PPG signals from volunteers at a sampling rate of 250 HZ, and the sampled text data file was saved in PC.

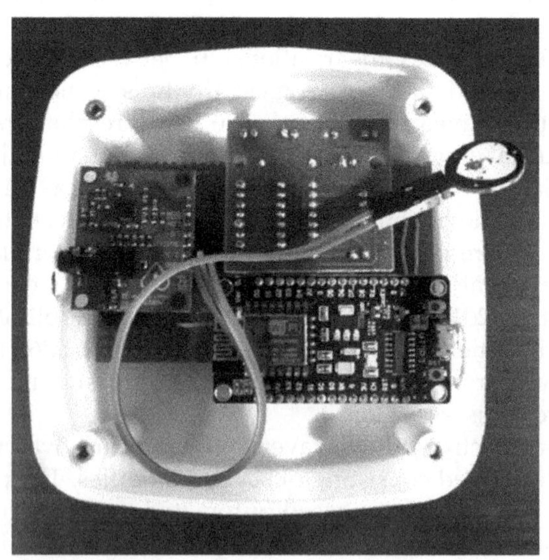

FIGURE 8.2
Indigenous PPG Signature Collection System.

8.3 Data Preprocessing

In order to minimize the impact of poor blood transmission through the peripheral tissues and motion artefact in the subsequent phases of the PPG signal for beat-to-beat estimation, a pre-conditioning of the signal is necessary. These steps are: (i) band-pass filtering (0.75 Hz to 8 Hz) to remove baseline drift and noise; (ii) automatic gain control (AGC) to limit the signal level; and (iii) signal smoothing and baseline-wandering removal.

Algorithm

I. Read sampled data value of PPG Signal (1000 to 4000 data points) with sampling frequency 250 Hz from PPG data points sensor module. Store the data points to an array variable.

II. Perform filtering of PPG waveform data for baseline and noise removal, using second-order Band Pass filter with lower cut-off frequency 0.75 Hz and upper cut-off frequency 8 Hz. (PPG signal is having the pulse wave frequency values in the range of 0.5–4.0 Hz.) Store the filtered data points to new array variable.

III. Compute the global maximum (MX) and minimum (MN) of all data points stored in the PPG array. Compute peak-to-peak value of PPG array.

IV. Compute the global maximum (MX1) and minimum (MN1) of all data points stored in filtered PPG array. Compute peak-to-peak value of filtered PPG array.

V. Set multiplying factor MF = (MX-MN)/(MX1-MN1). Multiply all data points in filtered PPG array by MF to adjust the gain.

8.4 Beat Extraction

The filtered PPG waveform sampled data are loaded into the array. The local minimal points, indicating the foot of PPG waveform points, are located in terms of index number, and the corresponding amplitudes are stored in two new arrays. The sampled data points between two successive index values form one complete beat of PPG. waveform. Thus, if there are N number of foots, the number of beats will be (N-1). The sampled data set of all beats is stored into a two-dimension array and in a data file "ppg_beat_matrix.txt."

Algorithm: Convert PPG waveform data into PPG beat matrix

Input: Read sampled data values from the "ppg_filtered.txt" file and store these values to array X.

Output: ppg_beat_matrix.txt

I. Find the local minimum (amplitude and sample no.) of all data points in array X and store in two arrays called min_peak and loc.
II. Find the size of the array min_peak and store to S.
III. K=(S-1), where K is number of beats (The sampled data points between two successive index values form one complete beat of PPG waveform. Thus, for N number of foots, there will be (N-1) beats).
IV. For i=1 to K.
V. Loc1=loc (i); Loc2=loc (i+1).
VI. N=(Loc2-Loc1) +1, where N is the number of sampled data points in a beat.
VII. For j=1 to N.
VIII. ppg_beat (J, I) = X(J,I).
IX. End for j.
X. End for i.
XI. Save ppg_beat to file "ppg_beat_matrix.txt."
XII. END

8.5 Fiducial Point Determination and Estimation of Clinical Parameters

Fiducial points of interest are the first and second derivatives of the PPG signal apart from the original PPG signal. Those fiducial points lead to the estimation of various clinical parameters revealing cardiac health/arterial aging, and so forth.

Algorithm:

Input: Read sampled data value of PPG waveform arranged beat-wise from file "ppg_beat_matrix.txt".

Read total number of beats: "B".

Output: PPG waveform fiducial points for all beats containing SP, STIME, DR, DRTIME, DP, DTIME, PTIME, SLP, DLP, PPGAI, M_PPI, M_PP_RATE.

I. For b (beat count) =1 to B.

II. Set S_SP(b), S_STIME(b), S_DPEAK(b), S_DRTIME(b), S_DP(b), S_DTIME(b), S_PTIME(b), S_SLP(b), S_DLP(b), S_PPGAI(b) to 0.

III. Store sampled data values to array variable "ppg_beat". Compute the size of array.

Compute first order derivative of all points stored in ppg_beat using formula: ppg_beat (i+1) – ppg_beat(i), where i is the sample no.

I. Store the values into array variable "ppg_derivative_1":

II. Compute second order derivative of all points stored in ppg_derivative_1 using formula: ppg_derivative_1(i+1)-ppg_derivative_1(i), where i is the sample no.

III. Store the values into array variable "ppg_derivative_2".

IV. Compute the length of array ppg_beat(i) and store it to N

V. Find maximum value or peak value and index of the array.

VI. Store peak value to variable "Systolic peak" and index to variable "peak time."

VII. Find zero crossing index of array ppg_derivative_1 and store to variable "Index_derivative_1".

VIII. Find zero crossing index of array ppg_derivative_2 and store to variable "Index_derivative_2".

IX. Compute the fiducial parameters as follows:

X.

- ✓ Systolic Peak: SP(b)=x(index_derivative_1(2))
- ✓ STIME(b)=index_derivative_1(2) *(1/250)
- ✓ Dicrotic notch: DR(b)=ppg_beat(index_derivative_2(2))
- ✓ DRTIME(b)=index_derivative_2(2) *(1/250)
- ✓ Diastolic Peak: DP(b)=ppg_beat(index_derivative_2(3))
- ✓ Diastolic Peak time: DTIME(b)=index_derivative_2(3)* (1/250)
- ✓ Pulse Time: PTIME(b)=Length of the array "X" *(1/250)
- ✓ Systolic Phase: SLP(b)=STIME(b)
- ✓ Distolic Phase: DLP(b)=DTIME(b)-STIME(b)
- ✓ Find negative peak index of array "index_derivative_2" and store it to array "A"

- ✓ The PPG augmented index: PPGAI(b)=(A(2)/SP)/(A(1)/SP)
- ✓ ppg_fiducial(b)=
  {SP(b), STIME(b), DR(b), DRTIME(b), DP(b), DTIME(b), PTIME(b), SLP(b), DLP(b), PPGAI(b)}
  End for b (beat count)**

XI. For b (beat count) =1 to B-1

XII. PPI(i)=STIME(i+1)-STIME(i)

XIII. PPI_RATE(i)=60/PPI(i)

End for b (beat count)**

Compute the mean values of SP, STIME, DR, DRTIME, DP, DTIME, PTIME, SLP, DLP and PPGAI, M_PPI, M_PP_RATE as follows:

$$M\_SP = \frac{1}{B}\sum_{j=1}^{B} SP(j)$$

$$M\_STIME = \frac{1}{B}\sum_{j=1}^{B} STIME(j)$$

$$M\_DR = \frac{1}{B}\sum_{j=1}^{B} DR(j)$$

$$M\_DRTIME = \frac{1}{B}\sum_{j=1}^{B} DRTIME(j)$$

$$M\_DP = \frac{1}{B}\sum_{j=1}^{B} DP(j)$$

$$M\_DTIME = \frac{1}{B}\sum_{j=1}^{B} DTIME(j)$$

$$M\_SLP = \frac{1}{B}\sum_{j=1}^{B} SLP(j)$$

$$M\_PTIME = \frac{1}{B}\sum_{j=1}^{B} PTIME(j)$$

$$M\_DLP = \frac{1}{B}\sum_{j=1}^{B} DLP(j)$$

$$M\_PPGAI = \frac{1}{B}\sum_{j=1}^{B} PPGAI(j)$$

$$M\_PPI = \frac{1}{B-1}\sum_{j=1}^{B-1} PPI(j)$$

$$SD\_PPI = \sqrt{\frac{1}{B-1}\sum_{j=1}^{B-1}\left(PPI(j) - M\_PPI\right)^2}$$

$$M\_PPI\_RATE = \frac{1}{B}\sum_{j=1}^{B-1} PPI\_RATE(j)$$

$$SD\_PPI\_RATE = \sqrt{\frac{1}{B-1}\sum_{j=1}^{B-1}\left(PPI\_RATE(j) - M\_PPI\_RATE\right)^2}$$

8.6 Estimation of HRV Parameters

8.6.1 Estimation of Time Domain HRV Parameters Using PPG Signal

PPG-based HRV parameter estimation is promising both in time and frequency domain. Monitoring may range from a minute to 24 hours. The standard deviation of the N-N interval in ECG signal (SDNN) values captured over 24 hours predict possible heart attack while SDNN values captured over 5 minutes are unable to do that [27]. The time domain HRV metrics include the SDPP, RMSSD, PP50, pPP50, HR Max – HR Min. The definitions [10] are as follows:

SDPP: The standard deviation in the P-P intermission (SDPP), that is, the square root of variance. A short-term 5-minute recording was chosen to find out SDPP. In the frequency domain, SDPP is correlated with various frequency band power and combined signal power. Longer recording periods reveal the human heart reacting to environmental impetus and also can catalogue the heart's response to various physiological processes. In ECG, the sympathetic nervous system (SNS) contributes to HRV [28]. Based on 24-hour monitoring, SDNN qualifiers state that the healthy heart reveals SDNN values above 100 ms, while an unhealthy heart falls below 50ms and ranges between 50 to 100 ms indicate conceded health [29].

RMSSD: The mean squared differences of successive PP intervals when raised to the power of ½ is RMSSD. The RMSSD is a prime measurement of HRV in time domain [30]. The RMSSD is identical to the metric SD1 in Poincaŕe plots and reflecting short-range heart-rate variability [30]. Long-interval RMSSD measurements are related to pNN50 and high frequency band power in frequency domain [31].

PP50: Interval differences between successive P-P intervals, which are greater than 50 ms.

pPP50: fraction of PP50 out of total number of PP intervals.

PP50, pPP50, and RMSSD are estimated using the interval between consecutive PP span. While depending on PP intermezzo changes, they remain unperturbed by inclinations in extended time series. Table 8.2 presents all the estimated time domain HRV parameters.

8.6.2 Estimation of Non-linear HRV Parameter Using PPG Signal

Poincaŕe plots were created by plotting the PP intermissions of a PPG signal as a function of itself delayed by one sample. Poincaŕe plots are helpful in erroneous detection of pulse propagations. Estimated non-linear HRV parameters [10] are as follows:

- SD1: Standard deviation in a Poincaré plot; perpendicular the line of identity.
- SD2: Standard deviation in a Poincaré plot; along the line of identity diagonal at the mean value of the data.

$$SD\,ratio = \frac{SD2}{SD1}$$

Table 8.2 also presents the non-linear HRV parameter. The SD ratio may be a new marker equivalent to PPGAI revealing vascular maturity (Vascular aging is associated with the failing mechanical and structural properties of the vascular wall leading to reduced arterial elasticity and compliance). The difference is that PPGAI was derived based on second-order derivative of PPG signal, but SD ratio is assessed here from filtered PPG signal. Figure 8.3 presents a distinctive Poincaŕe plot of 38-year-old subject.

Algorithm:

Input: Read sampled data value of PPG waveform arranged beat wise from file "ppg_beat_matrix.txt" and store these to array "X".

Read number of sampled data, L.

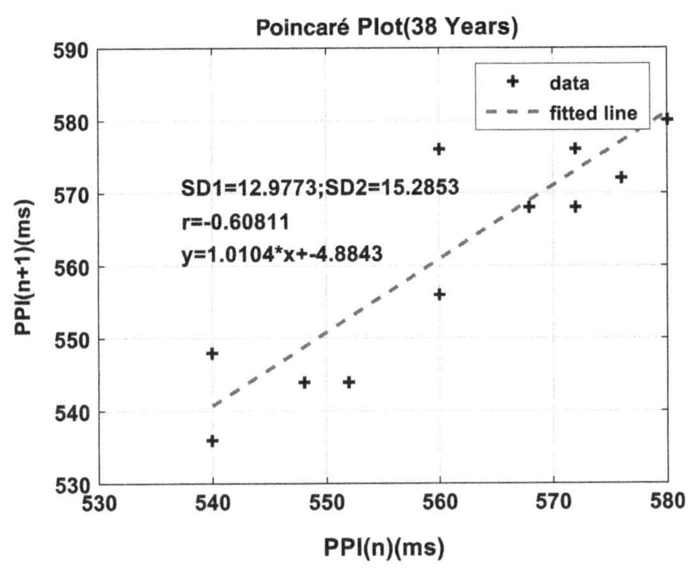

FIGURE 8.3
Poincaŕe Plot of 38-year-old Subject.

Output: SDNN RMSSD PP50, pPP50 MEAN SD1 SD2.

I. Store the L no. of sampled data to array ppg.
II. Find maximum value or peak value and index of the array (peak, index).
III. No. of beats (B) =peak-1.
IV. For i=1 to B-1.
V. ppi(i)=(loc(i+1)-loc(i)) *1000.
VI. end of loop
VII. $mean\_ppi = \frac{1}{B-1}\sum_{i=1}^{B-1} ppi(i)$
VIII. $SDNN = \sqrt{\frac{1}{B-1}\sum_{i=1}^{B-1}\left(ppi(i) - mean\_ppi\right)^2}$
IX. PP50=0
X. For i=1 to B-1
XI. Heart_rate=(ppi(i+1)-ppi(i))*1000
XII. If abs((ppi(i+1)-ppi(i))) *1000>=50
XIII. PP50=PP50+1
XIV. end of loop

XV. end of loop

XVI. $mean\,of\,heart\,rate_m = \frac{1}{B-1}\sum_{i=1}^{B-1} heart\_rate(i)$

XVII. $SDNN = \sqrt{\frac{1}{B-1}\sum_{i=1}^{B-1} (heart\_rate(i) - rate_m)^2}$

XVIII. For i=1 to B-1

XIX. X(i)=ppi(i); Y(i)=ppi(i+1)

XX. end of loop

XXI. Scatter Plot X vs Y

XXII. Find best fit line using X and Y arrays to compute C and m such that linear equation $Y = mX + C$ is formed.

XXIII. $mean, X_m = \frac{1}{B-1}\sum_{i=1}^{B-1} X_i$; $mean, Y_m = \frac{1}{B-1}\sum_{i=1}^{B-1} Y_i$

XXIV. $SD1 = \sqrt{\frac{1}{B-1}\sum_{I=1}^{B-1}(X_i - X_m)^2}$; $SD2 = \sqrt{\frac{1}{B-1}\sum_{i=1}^{B-1}(Y_i - Y_m)^2}$

XXV. Compute correlation coefficient of Poincaŕe as follows:

$$r_{XY} = \frac{\sum_{i=1}^{B-1}(X_i - X_m)(Y_i - Y_m)}{\sqrt{\sum_{i=1}^{B-1}(X_i - X_m)^2 \sum_{i=1}^{B-1}(Y_i - Y_m)^2}}$$

XXVI. End of algorithm

8.7 Results and Discussions

The fiducial points of 15 subjects as systolic peak and time, dicrotic notch peak and time, diastolic peak and time, systolic and diastolic phase durations, pulse interval, PPGAI, and instant heart rate variability values are determined in this study. The mean values of all these parameters (over 10 beats) are determined for each subject. The average values over 15 subjects are estimated (Table 8.1). Table 8.2 presents the time domain PPG-based and non-linear HRV parameters.

Two main phases representing the cardiac cycle are *systole* and *diastole*, and they track each other in order. The diastolic phase begins with the relaxation of heart muscles when blood returns to the heart and begins to fill the atria and ventricles. A signal then triggers to the sinoatrial node to induce contraction

TABLE 8.1

Fiducial Parameters and Clinical Index Determination Using PPG and SDPPG Signal

SL NO.	YRS	M_STIME	M_SYSTOLIC	M_DRTIME	M_DR	M_DTIME	M_DIASTOL	M_PAI	M_SLP	M_DLP	M_PPI	M_PP_RATE
1	62	0.1664	2.1023	0.2604	1.2416	0.4948	0.0985	0.1101	0.1664	0.3284	0.496	121.1297
2	57	0.1688	1.7068	0.2372	1.3537	0.4892	0.0678	0.1210	0.1688	0.3204	0.4876	123.0706
3	55	0.1776	2.159	0.2568	1.334	0.5476	0.2177	0.1602	0.1776	0.37	0.548	109.5617
4	51	0.184	2.1522	0.2584	1.5072	0.6352	0.0041	0.0115	0.184	0.4512	0.6352	94.5655
5	50	0.328	1.305	0.4006	1.0147	0.6303	0.481	0.1721	0.328	0.3023	0.6423	94.7909
6	40	0.1692	1.9932	0.2564	1.3983	0.652	0.0692	0.4847	0.1692	0.4828	0.65	92.3381
7	38	0.1512	2.1937	0.2236	1.6813	0.5748	0.2681	0.1528	0.1512	0.4236	0.5756	104.2609
8	36	0.19	2.0546	0.2708	1.6047	0.6412	0.2798	0.5031	0.19	0.4512	0.6352	94.6073
9	35	0.1248	1.5463	0.1804	1.238	0.4448	0.5681	0.4227	0.1248	0.32	0.4448	134.95
10	25	0.1604	2.1316	0.2428	1.1415	0.5328	0.0943	0.4091	0.1604	0.3724	0.5332	112.5634
11	23	0.1668	1.9932	0.2336	1.5586	0.5348	0.1214	0.2234	0.1668	0.368	0.5352	112.1696
12	22	0.1716	2.2488	0.2748	1.4592	0.6576	0.0304	0.3013	0.1716	0.486	0.6568	91.3675
13	21	0.1528	3.3274	0.2356	2.4229	0.584	0.6296	0.3598	0.1528	0.4312	0.5844	102.793
14	12	0.1716	2.1598	0.2748	1.4014	0.6576	0.0292	0.3013	0.1716	0.486	0.6568	91.3675
15	11	0.1496	1.9933	0.2216	1.5485	0.4472	0.3003	0.0914	0.1496	0.2976	0.4468	134.4152

M_STIME	Mean Systolic Peak time (s)
M_SYSTOLIC	Mean Systolic Peak amplitude (Volt)
M_DRTIME	Mean Dicrotic time (s)
M_DR	Mean Dicrotic Peak amplitude (Volt)
M_DTIME	Mean Diastolic Peak time (s)
M_DIASTOL	Mean Diastolic Peak amplitude (Volt)
M_PAI	Mean PPG augmentation index
M_SLP	Mean Systolic phase duration (s)
M_DLP	Mean Diastolic phase duration (s)
M_PPI	Mean pulse to pulse interval (s)
M_PP_RATE	Mean instantaneous heart rate (bpm)

TABLE 8.2

HRV Parameters for 15 Volunteers from Their Extracted PPG Signals

SL NO.	YRS	BEATS	SDPP ±ms	RMSSD ±ms	pPP50 %	SD1 ms	SD2 ms
1	62	31	17.407	14.689	20	16.047	18.983
2	57	32	11.376	11.335	9.68	10.401	12.393
3	55	28	11.045	16.788	25.92	13.421	8.5163
4	50	25	11.517	13.946	45.83	13.297	10.739
5	51	24	25.075	29.252	52.17	23.661	27.314
6	40	24	15.421	18.175	30.44	14.316	16.837
7	38	27	13.633	10.423	7.78	12.977	15.285
8	36	26	35.516	28.902	39.13	37.468	34.979
9	35	33	29.748	18.735	21.87	33.329	27.634
10	22	24	31.734	36.171	47.83	31.326	33.268
11	21	27	29.483	29.296	46.15	29.369	30.134
12	23	29	25.515	18.333	25.0	23.970	26.966
13	25	29	12.212	11.748	10.71	12.123	12.859
14	12	24	31.734	36.171	47.82	31.326	33.268
15	11	35	25.177	13.349	20.58	23.711	25.228

in atria allowing blood leaving it. Another wave of contraction commences as ventricular systole contracts insisted the aortic and pulmonary valves to open. For a typical heart rate of 75 beats per minute (bpm), the cardiac cycle requires 0.8 sec to complete the cycle. The diastolic phase time (M_DLP) is always greater that systolic phase time (M_SLP) as is evident from Table 8.1 for all the subjects.

Diastolic phase is the time period when most of the coronary perfusion occurs, hence reduced diastolic phase time creates poor circulation of blood. At a particular heart rate (bpm), there is ratio of systolic phase time to diastolic phase time, which is a diagnostic measure. Increase of which indicates diastolic dysfunction. It is pertinent to mention that. Myocardial ischemia occurs when blood flowing to the heart muscle (myocardium) is being obstructed by a partial or complete blockage of a coronary artery. Prolonged myocardial ischemia generated out of diastolic dysfunction may lead to the myocardial infraction or heart attack.

Subjects having lower values of PPGAI (as per our definition), are very prone to cardiac artery disease. (51 year-old and 11-year old subjects as per Table 8.1 are showing M_PAI values of 0.0115 and 0.0914 respectively). Table 8.1 also reveals that systolic peak (Volts) is always higher than diastolic peak and the dicrotic notch peak is in between the systolic and diastolic peaks. The peak-to-peak distance in successive PPG beats varies within 0.44±0.22 s.

Table 8.2 presents the time domain and non-linear HRV parameters. Figure 8.3 represents the correlation between short-term and long-term variability of the PPG signal with its one-time instant lagged signal for a

38-year-old subject. The SDPP, RMSSD, pPP50 parameters vary from subject to subject without a gross variation in heart rate variability. The dependence of SDPP on length of recording needs to be studied. $SD\,ratio = \frac{SD2}{SD1}$ like PPGAI assesses vascular health or atherosclerosis lower SD ratio (as per our definition) indicated healthy vascular status. The long-term variability SD2 in the Poincaré plot may act as an independent prognostic variable. The Poincaré plot, may be considered as time-series data where auto correlation is found among successive/lagged sample points. This auto-correlation behavior in a time series is a signature of its memory and significant from a diagnostic point of view of cognitive diseases. The greater the correlation coefficient (r) in a Poincaré plot, the less facile the situation from the disease-control point of view. In the absence of much physiological /clinical interpretation in Poincaré plots, it becomes a statistical way of inferencing from time-series data. We have also assumed that the variabilities SD1 and SD2 vary linearly, which requires that the variation of SD1 and SD2 varies linearly is to be supported clinically.

8.8 Conclusion

The present work required some effort to explain the role of the fiducial parameters in explaining cardiac health and heart rate variability using a PPG signal. The indigenous hardware, detail signal processing and characteristic parameter determination algorithms are the contribution of the presented research effort. Heart-rate variability parameters in time domain and non-linear domain were also estimated from the collected PPG signals. This work can be further enhanced by making an extended database followed by machine learning based automated classification system among persons with normal and diagnosed cardiac and respiratory abnormalities. The frequency domain HRV parameters from the PPG signal collected over extended period of time are expected to enhance the quality of the database leading to better applicability in diagnostics.

Acknowledgments

The authors are grateful to Jadavpur University, Calcutta, and the National Institute of Technology Rourkela for supporting the research.

References

1. Moraes, Jermana L., Matheus X. Rocha, Glauber G. Vasconcelos, José E. Vasconcelos Filho, Victor Hugo C. de Albuquerque, & Auzuir R. Alexandria (2018). Advances in photopletysmography signal analysis for biomedical applications. *Sensors*, 18: 1894.
2. Kundu, Madhusree, Palash Kundu, & Seshu Kumar Damarla (2017). *A chemometric approach to monitoring: Product quality assessment, process fault detection and miscellaneous applications*, CRC Press. (www.crcpress.com/Chemometric-Monitoring-Product-Quality-Assessment-Process-Fault-Detection/Kundu-Kundu-Damarla/p/book/9781498780070).
3. Hertzman, A. B. (1938). The blood supply of various skin areas as estimated by the photoelectric plethysmograph. American Journal of Physiology, 124: 328–340.
4. Nabeel. P. M., & Jayaraj, J. (2017). Single-source PPG based local pulse wave velocity measurement: A potential cuffless blood pressure estimation technique. *Physiological Measurement*, 38: 2122–2140.
5. Oppenheim, M. J. & Sittig, D. F. (1995). An innovative dicrotic notch detection algorithm which combines rule-based logic with digital signal processing techniques. *Computers and Biomedical Research*, 28(2): 154–170.
6. Gonzalez, R., Manzo, A., Delgado, J., Padilla, J. M., & Trenor, B. (2008). A computer based photoplethysmographic vascular analyzer through derivatives. *Computers in Cardiology*, 35: 177–180.
7. Chan, G. S. H., Paul, M. M., Branko, G. C., Lu, W., & Nigel, H. L. (2007). Automatic detection of left ventricular ejection time from a finger photoplethysmographic pulse oximetry waveform: Comparison with Doppler aortic measurement. Physiological Measurement. (28): 1–14.
8. Allen, J. (2007). Photoplethysmography and its application in clinical physiological measurement. *Physiological Measurement*, 28: RI–R39.
9. F. Shaffer & J. P. Ginsberg (2017). An overview of heart rate variability metrics and norms. *Front Public Health*, 5: 258 (doi: 10.3389/fpubh.2017.00258).
10. Hon, E. H., & Lee, S. T. (1965). Electronic evaluations of the fetal heart rate patterns preceding fetal death, further observations. American Journal of Obstetrics & Gynecology, 87: 814–826.
11. Kleiger, R. E., Miller, J. P., Bigger, J. T., Moss, A. J., & the Multi-center Post-Infarction Research Group (1987). Decreased heart rate variability and its association with increased mortality after acute myocardial infarction. American Journal of Cardiology, 59: 256–262.
12. Malik, M., Farrell, T., Cripps, T., & Camm, A. J. (1989). Heart rate variability in relation to prognosis after myocardial infarction: Selection of optimal processing techniques. *European Heart Journal*, 10: 1060–1074.
13. Bigger, J. T., Fleiss, J. L., Steinman, R. C., Rolnitzky, L. M., Kleiger, R. E., & Rottman, J. N. (1992). Frequency domain measures of heart period variability and mortality after myocardial infarction. *Circulation*, 85: 164–171.
14. Bhowmick, Subhajit, Palash Kumar Kundu & Dharma Das Mandal (2020). HRV performance analysis in photoplethysmography and electrocardiography. In: The proceedings of the IEEE (CALCON 2020).

15. Kuusela, T. (2013). Methodological aspects of heart rate variability analysis. In: Kamath, M. V., Watanabe, M. A., & Upton, A. R. M. (eds.). *Heart Rate Variability (HRV) Signal Analysis*. Boca Raton, FL: CRC Press, pp. 9–42.
16. Selvaraj, N., Jaryal, A., Santhosh, J., Deepak, K. K. & Anand, S. (2008). Assessment of heart rate variability derived from finger-tip photoplethysmography as compared to electrocardiography. *Journal of Medical Engineering & Technology*, 32(6): 479–484.
17. Johnston, W. & Mendelson, Y., (2005). Extracting heart rate variability from a wearable reflectance pulse oximeter. Proceedings of the IEEE 31st Annual Northeast Bioengineering Conference, Hoboken, NJ: 157–158.
18. Task Force of the European Society of Cardiology and The North American Society of Pacing and Electrophysiology (1996). Heart rate variability: Standards of measurement, physiological interpretation, and clinical use. *European Heart Journal*, 17: 354–381.
19. Elgendi, Mohamed, Richard Fletcher, Yongbo Liang1, Newton Howard, Nigel H. Lovell, Derek Abbott, Kenneth Lim, & Rabab Ward (2019). The use of photoplethysmography for assessing hypertension, *Nature Partner Journal, Digital Medicine*, 2: 60.
20. Bolanos, M., Nazeran, H., & Haltiwanger (2006). Comparison of heart rate variability signal features derived from electrocardiography and photoplethysmography in healthy individuals. Proceedings of the 28th IEEE EMBS Annual International Conference, New York, Aug 30–Sept 3, pp. 4289–4294.
21. Subasi, Abdulhamit (2019). *Practical guide for biomedical signals analysis using machine learning techniques, A MATLAB based approach*. Academic Press, pp. 27–87.
22. Khan, Emroz, Forsad Al Hossain, Shiekh Zia Uddin, & Kamrul Hasan (2015). A robust heart rate monitoring scheme using photoplethysmographic signals corrupted by intense motion artifacts, *IEEE Transactions on Biomedical Engineering*, 63(3): 1–10.
23. Mani, A. R., Mazloom, R., Haddadian, Z., & Montagnese, S. (2018). Body temperature fluctuation analysis in cirrhosis. *Liver* International, 38: 378–379. doi: 10.1111/liv.13539.
24. Hsu, C.-H., Tsai, M.-Y., Huang, G.-S., Lin, T.-C., Chen, K.-P., Ho, S.-T., et al. (2012). Poincaré plot indexes of heart rate variability detect dynamic autonomic modulation during general anesthesia induction. *Acta Anaesthesiol. Taiwan*, 50: 12–18. doi: 10.1016/J.AAT.2012.03.002.
25. Satti, Reem, Noor-U/-Hoda Abid, Matteo Bottaro, Michele De Rui, Maria Garrido, Mohammad R. Raoufy, Sara Montagnese & Ali R. Mani (2019). The application of the extended Poincare Plot in the analysis of physiological variabilities frontiers in physiology. 10, Article 116.
26. Shaffer, F., McCraty, R., & Zerr, C. L. (2014). A healthy heart is not a metronome: An integrative review of the heart's anatomy and heart rate variability, Frontiers in Psychology, 5: 1040.10.3389/fpsyg.2014.01040.
27. Grant, C. C., van Rensburg, D. C., Strydom, N., and Viljoen, M. (2011) Importance of tachogram length and period of recording during noninvasive investigation of the autonomic nervous system. *Ann Noninvasive Electrocardiol*, 16: 131–9.10.1111/j.1542-474X.2011.00422.x.

28. Kleiger, R. E., Miller, J. P., Bigger, J. T., Jr, & Moss, A. J. (1987). Decreased heart rate variability and its association with increased mortality after acute myocardial infarction. American Journal of Cardiology, 59: 256–262.10.1016/0002-9149(87)90795-8.
29. Ciccone, A. B., Siedlik, J. A., Wecht, J. M., Deckert, J. A., Nguyen, N. D., & Weir, J. P. (2017). RMSSD and SD1 are identical heart rate variability metrics. *Muscle Nerve*, 10.1002/mus.25573.
30. Fei, L., Copie, X., Malik, M., & Camm, A. J. (1996). Short- and long-term assessment of heart rate variability for risk stratification after acute myocardial infarction. American Journal of Cardiology, 77: 681–4.10.1016/S0002-9149(97)89199-0.
31. Shirazi, A. H., Raoufy, M. R., Ebadi, H., De Rui, M., Schiff, S., Mazloom, R., et al. (2013). Quantifying memory in complex physiological time-series. Public Library of Science *One*, 8: e72854. doi: 10.1371/journal.pone.0072854

9

ARIMA Prediction Model Based Forecasting for COVID-19 Infected and Recovered Cases

Tamoghna Mukherjee, Sudarshan Nandy, Akshay Vinayak, and Simran Kumari

CONTENTS

9.1 Introduction

The COVID-19 outbreak was confirmed on 31 December 2019, when China reported to the World Health Organization a cluster of pneumonia cases from an unidentified cause in Wuhan City, Hubei Province. [1] The virus is referred to as SARS-CoV-2, which caused the disease COVID-19, then spread to other provinces in China and around the world and is termed a pandemic. India witnessed a COVID-19 outbreak in late January 2020, and the nation recorded more than 2.91 million confirmed COVID-19 cases and more than 54,000 deaths by August 2020. In this case, effective COVID-19 prediction plays a very important role in the fight against corona virus and, based on this forecast, social rules are defined, such as lock-down times.

In view of this scenario, the researcher proposes different estimation approaches to approximate the nearly exact number of cases that have been infected and recovered. Given the present situation, there is an urgent need to monitor and forecast the frequency of COVID-19 to handle this epidemic more precisely. Time series models may play a key role in predicting the impact of the COVID-19 pandemic and can suggest necessary measures in resolving the situation [5]. The COVID-19 forecast has played an important role in recognizing the threat of contamination and the crucial rate of duplication. These forecasts would help to boost policy implantation to strengthen health sector capability and implement social distance measures across India [7–9]. Developing efficient models of momentary forecasting helps one to know the number of probable cases [2].

Based on various factors and assumptions, possible biases are imposed on the mathematical models [3]. The forecasting process is an error-driven iterative methodology composed of four distinct phases: forecast data collection, possible forecast model compilation, provisional forecast model estimation of parameters and diagnostic power. A brief look at the data structure and trend characteristics should be added after collecting the data and identifying the forecasting query to find a fitting model. If a model has been established, it will then be diagnostically tested against the historical data to determine if the time series is represented correctly. For example, the analysis in the Auto-Regressive Integrated Moving Average (ARIMA) model involves testing the residuals between the forecast and the actual series and deciding if they are minimal, randomly distributed and uncorrelated, and whether the chosen model is assumed to be a good match.

The ARIMA technique is a mathematical approach to evaluate and create a predictive model that better describes a time series by modelling the data associations. A variety of benefits of the ARIMA model have been found in observational studies that endorse the ARIMA as an effective way to predict especially short-term time series. Using its purely statistical approach, the ARIMA method only includes previous data from a time series to generalize the prediction. Therefore, the ARIMA method would improve forecast accuracy while reducing parameter counts. Also named Box-Jenkins (after the original authors), ARIMA is generally superior to the exponential smoothing strategies because the sample is comparatively long and the relation between past observations is constant. Various paradigms achieve variation in various types of time-series.

First Order DLM performs well in annual data while ARIMA operates well for other and quarterly data. ANNs delivers a pleasing performance in forecasting monthly results. It has been observed that statistically sophisticated paradigms, such as ANNs, are likely to deliver greater prediction precision in monthly time series than do simplistic paradigms. Duration of the time series determines the usefulness of ANNs. The main reasons why the ANNs displays so much variation are seen in various categorical time series, since the prediction performance of the ANNs depends on how much historical information is available for the training process. The more evidence that was provided in the past, the more accurate the predictions became.

Finally, complex DLM models do not require more than basic DLM models in forecasting. The tendency is mirrored in all-time series forecasting. One inference is that forecast success depends on the longitude of the forecast horizon. The degree of predictive uncertainty usually increases as the horizon is raised, but there is some absence in ANNs where the model isn't robust. The strongest ARIMA model has proved effective in short-term forecasting for mid-length time series. It also has the potential to capture seasonal trends in time sequence. When the time series is short and has no seasonal history, a first order DLM algorithm is suggested for short-term forecasting. The first order DLM offers a predictive model that's simple, fast, reliable and precise. A well-designed ANNs, also with seasonal variations at all prediction horizons, demonstrates strong success in long-time series forecasting.

In limited/short training performances, ANNs have low efficiency. This shows that a large number of samples are needed by the ANNs used in this work to achieve a reliable and rational forecast outcome. When using the ANNs in time series forecasting, forecasters should always be mindful of the calculation time spent during the training process. Construction of computationally capable and practical models is highly necessary so that they can support decision makers, medical professionals and even the general public. It will help the medical system get ready for the new patients by modelling the disease and offering potential estimates of the probable numbers of regular events. Models of mathematical analysis are useful to both estimate and monitor the epidemic's global hazard. Within this project, we used the ARIMA model to estimate the occurrence of COVID-19 disease.

The remainder of the chapter is structured according to the following: Section 9.2 consists of a summary of the associated articles by literature. Section 9.3 describes the data selection, model creation, and results achieved for COVID-19 forecasting for the Indian states of Delhi, West Bengal, Tamil Nadu and Maharashtra and addresses the predictive results in Section 9.4. The chapter ends with a conclusion and summary in Section 9.5.

9.2 Literature Review

The emerging global pandemic known as COVID-19 infection requires diverse methodologies for monitoring and anticipating adverse consequences. COVID-19 daily cases in Canada, France, India, South Korea were forecasted by a novel hybrid model ARIMA-WBF for COVID-19 prediction [1].

Regression modeling was applied in another analysis to predict COVID-19 population cases in Brazil. The investigators adopted evidence from ten countries with a high occurrence of COVID-19. Models for multi-step forecasting were tested. Out-of-sample prediction errors of less than 6.9 percent were achieved by the best models. The most effective methods for forecasting

COVID-19 cases in the scenarios tested were SVR and stacking ensemble [2]. Another idea was a basic econometric model that could be useful in forecasting COVID-2019 spread. The Auto Regressive Integrated Moving Average (ARIMA) model estimates the occurrence and frequency of COVID-19 epidemiological data from Johns Hopkins University.

Logarithmic transformation is achieved in assessing the influence of seasonality on prediction. The autocorrelation function (ACF) and partial autocorrelation function (PACF) data correlogram has demonstrated that both the frequency and occurrence of COVID-2019 are not affected by the seasonality [3]. A data-driven model is also useful for forecasting recorded and recovered cases in Italy after the country had been locked down for 60 days. COVID-19 cumulative patient data from the Italian Ministry of Health website covers cases reported and retrieved from mid-February to the end of March. It has introduced a seasonal ARIMA prediction package with a predictive model R. Predictions were made for reported case models with 93.75 percent accuracy and 84.4 percent accuracy for recovered case models. Predictions were for 182,757 untreated patients, and that treated cases could number 81,635 at the end of May [4]. Developing an Auto-Regressive Integrated Moving Average (ARIMA) model to predict COVID-19's epidemiological trend in Italy, Spain and France – the most affected countries in Europe – provided some new insights. From February 2020 to April 2020, the regular prevalence data for COVID-19 were retrieved from the WHO website.

Several ARIMA models have been developed from this data, with different ARIMA parameters. For Italy, Spain and France, ARIMA models (0,2,1), ARIMA models (1,2,0) and ARIMA models (0,2,1) with the lowest MAPE values (4,7520, 5,8486 and 5,6335) were chosen as best models. This research suggested that the ARIMA models are useful for future COVID-19 prevalence prediction [5]. Interestingly, the prediction of SutteARIMA's short-term use of recorded COVID-19 and IBEX cases in Spain provided some new results. Authenticated Spanish COVID-19 data was obtained from Yahoo Finance, from Worldometer and Spain Stock Exchange data (IBEX 35). In this review the SutteARIMA method was used. The researchers applied predictive precision tests for the assessment of the forecasting processes, mean absolute percentage error (MAPE).

Based on the findings of the forecasting methods ARIMA and SutteARIMA, it was hypothesized that the SutteARIMA approach is better suited to estimating the regular forecasts of reported cases of COVID-19 and IBEX in Spain [6]. A particular model for prediction was developed to deal with cases in India. The study indicates an upward trajectory in the days ahead for those cases. An assessment of the time series also shows an exponential growth in the number of instances. Time series study indicates an exponential rise in infected cases. However, interventions such as lockdowns are also likely to affect this forecast, and cases will begin to decline after approximately one month [7]. In the coming days, predictions on certain trajectories were made in India associated with COVID-19 using the Autoregression

Integrated Moving Average Model (ARIMA) and Richard's algorithm. They expected a total of 197 deaths (95 It is clear from the above discussions that the forecasting models as mentioned would play a significant role in curbing the epidemic, and ARIMA is one of the most enhanced models that plays a key role in precise forecasting).

Model assessment approach based on mathematical analysis suggests the validity of the model selected [8]. A thoughtful idea of using exponential and classic models of susceptible-infected-recovered (SIR) based on the available data to render daily short and long-term predictions is also proposed. Based on the SIR model, it is projected that by the end of May 2020 India would reach equilibrium with a final epidemic size of around 13,000. However, if India reaches the group transmission point, the calculation will be invalid. The effect of social distancing is also measured by comparing data from various geographical areas, once again with the presumption of no group transmission [9].

A novel approach to systematize ongoing activities in the area of data science was also carried out. As well as reviewing the increasingly growing body of recent studies, surveying public databases and repositories that can be used to monitor COVID-19 spread and mitigation strategies for further study was accomplished. A bibliometric study of the papers published in this short span of time as part of that survey was provided. Ultimately, building on these observations, illustration was made of rising obstacles and pitfalls that were found in the works being surveyed. A live resource repository was also created for keeping updated with the latest resources, including new papers and datasets [10]. In another study a summary of AI and Big Data was produced, describing the applications in COVID-19 combat, and then highlighting problems and concerns relevant to state-of-the-art solutions.

The study noted that the AI-based approach is highly appropriate to minimize the effects of the COVID-19 pandemic, as large quantities of COVID-19 data are becoming accessible thanks to various technologies and efforts. The AI experiments are not applied on a broad scale and/or clinically validated, but they are nevertheless beneficial because they can provide medical personnel and policymakers with a quick response and useful secret knowledge [11].

9.3 Proposed Method

9.3.1 Data Collection

We relied on daily data for four Indian states, that is, reported and recovered cases: Delhi, Maharashtra, Tamil Nadu and West Bengal. The data was collected from Health Ministry, Government of India. Both these databases were obtained during the national lock-down and unlocking phases over a period of four-and-a-half months from March to August 2020. A practical approach was pursued in which it was conjectured the trajectory would be continuous. We followed time series forecasting methods through the application of ARIMA methodology to forecast reported COVID-19 events.

9.3.2 Auto Regressive Integrated Moving Average

The approach is a collection of models that defines a given infographic related to its previous data, which consists of lags and lagged prediction inaccuracies, for the purpose of using the equation to predict later data.

- AR: Autoregression. This term defines an approach that utilizes the dependent connection between a consideration and few lagged considerations.
- I: Integrated. The use of difference of fresh considerations for making the collected data stationary.
- MA: Moving Average. This calculation uses the reliance of an consideration with a remaining inaccuracy from a moving average model applied to lagged considerations.

An ARIMA model consists of three parameters: p, d, q, as described below:

- p – refers to auto-regressive component order,
- q – refers to the order of the typical movable component,
- d – refers to the number of differentiation steps.

AR and MA Model, A pure Auto Regressive (AR only) model, is one where X_t depends only on its own lags. That is, X_t is a function of the "lags of X_t."

$$X_t = \alpha + \beta_1 X_{t-1} + \beta_2 X_{t-2} + \ldots\ldots + \beta_p X_{t-p} + \varepsilon_1 \quad (1)$$

where, X_{t-1} is the lag1 of the series, beta1 is the coefficient of lag1 that the model estimates and alpha is the intercept term, also estimated by the model. Likewise, a pure Moving Average (MA only) model is one where X_t depends only on the lagged forecast errors.

$$X_t = \alpha + \varepsilon_t + \varphi_1 \varepsilon_{t-1} + \varphi_2 \varepsilon_{t-2} + \ldots + \varphi_q \varepsilon_{t-q} \quad (2)$$

where the error terms are the errors of the auto-regressive models of the respective lags.

The errors ε_t and ε_{t-1} are the errors from the following equations:

$$X_t = \beta_1 X_{t-1} + \beta_2 X_{t-2} + \ldots + \beta_0 X_0 + \varepsilon_t \quad (3)$$

$$X_{t-1} = \beta_1 X_{t-2} + \beta_2 X_{t-3} + \ldots + \beta_0 X_0 + \varepsilon_{t-1} \quad (4)$$

An ARIMA model is one where the time series is separated to keep it stationary at least once, and you add the words AR and MA. So the equation becomes:

$$X_t = \alpha + \beta_1 X_{t-1} + \beta_2 X_{t-2} + \ldots. + \beta_p X_{t-p}\ \varepsilon_t + \varphi_1 \varepsilon_{t-1} + \varphi_2 \varepsilon_{t-2} + \ldots + \varphi_q \varepsilon_{t-q} \quad (5)$$

ARIMA model in words:

Predicted X_t = Constant + Linear combination Lags of X (up to p lags) + Linear

Combination of Lagged forecast errors (up to q lags) Therefore, the purpose is to define the p, d and q values. The method comprises six phases, as seen below:

Step 1: If a time series has a portion of pattern or seasonality, then it must be stationary before we can estimate using ARIMA.

Step 2: If the time series is not stationary, it has to be made stationary stationarized by distinction. Find the first discrepancy and then measure whether it is stationary. We may take as many different distinctions as we can. We will need to ensure the seasonal variations research is completed.

Step 3: Checking the model's accuracy is required. Validation of split train search shall be included.

Step 4: By using ACF and PACF to decide if AR(s), MA(s), or both must be used.

Step 5: Create the model and limit the number of forecast times to N (depends on your needs).

Step 6: The values expected are correlated with the real observations in the validation study.

The method builds an ARIMA model to predict the linear components of the disease time series and produces a collection of out-of-sample forecasts.

9.4 Experimental Results and Discussion

To suit a model with ARIMA, we first define model parameters. We will determine the value of the model's parameters using ACF plot and PACF plot. For each training dataset, the "best" fitted ARIMA model is selected using AIC and BIC values. For the input dataset the fitted ARIMA models are ARIMA (2,2,2), where p=2, q=2 and d=2 respectively. As the ARIMA model is installed, forecasts for the input dataset of each state are created from the month of March 2020 to December 2020. We developed individual predictions for confirmed and recovered cases four months out, based on the methodology described in this report. Figures 9.1, 9.3, 9.5 and 9.7 reflect stationary data of the cases observed for each condition. Figures 9.2, 9.4, 9.6 and 9.8 reflect the forecasted time series of each state's stationary datasets as determined via the ARIMA model. If the actual values are obtained for the state-wise COVID-19 cases in India and other countries, our model can be conveniently updated on a regular or periodic basis. The study on the COVID-19 data for Delhi, West Bengal, Tamil Nadu and Maharashtra is presented. It also introduces the topic of ARIMA model-based forecasting.

ARIMA Model Based analysis for Delhi: The main sequence analysis ACF and PACF plots revealed that the series was not stationary. Modifications allowed the series transition to reach stationary. After distribution of the differentiated sequence ACF and PACF, an ARIMA model (2,2,2) was established.

In order to validate the adequacy of the model, the Normalized Bayesian Knowledge Criterion (BIC) has been analysed. Again, the ARIMA (2,2,2) model was found to be the most suitable model with the Normalized BIC value of 13,171 for the recovered model and 11,589 for the verified model within a class of substantially adequate ARIMA (p, d, q) models with the same dataset (Table 9.1). According to the Stationary R-squared definition, a positive R-squared means that the one to be considered is better than the reference one, which is true in this case, so we should conclude that it is a stronger one. In another finding on the Normalized Bayesian Knowledge Criterion (BIC), it was observed that in a class of statistically valid ARIMA models (p, d, q) fitting the sequence, the ARIMA model (0,0,0) had the BIC value of 20.197 for the retrieved model and 20.059 for the verified model, which is far higher than our current ARIMA model (2,2,2) and, thus, we may infer that the existing equipped model is sufficient. A prediction as depicted in Figure 9.2 was rendered based on the above observation. The following observations were made from the forecasted data: (1) In the projected dataset for recovered cases, the maximum number of cases will be reported in the first week of November 2020, while the detected cases will be the lowest as compared with the highest number of cases in the last week of December 2020. (2) In the projected dataset for confirmed cases, the maximum number of cases will be reported in the first week of October 2020, while the detected cases will be the lowest as opposed to the highest number of cases in the last week of December 2020.

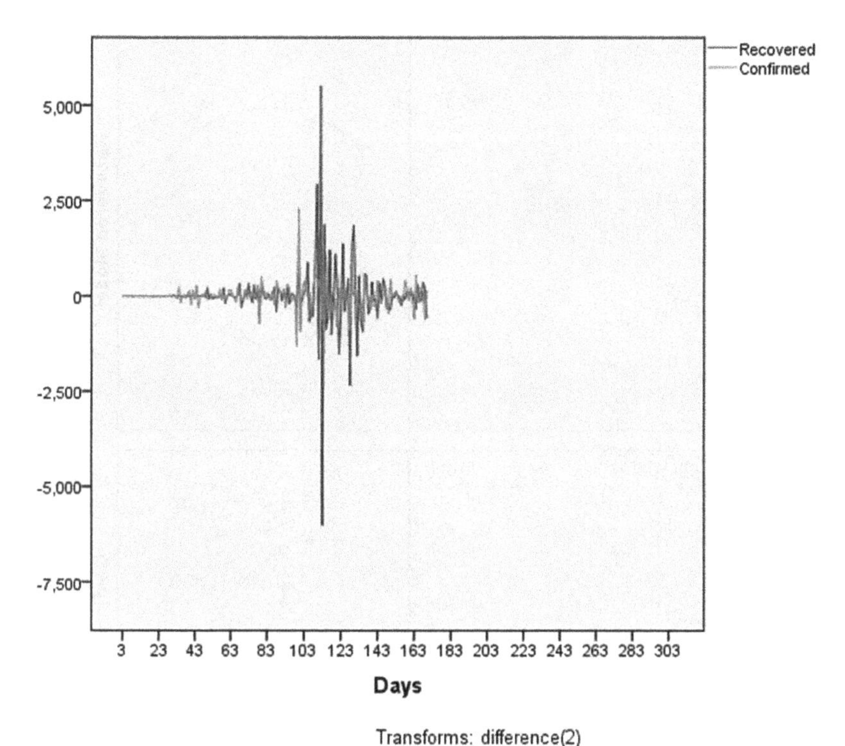

FIGURE 9.1
Sequence Plot for the State of Delhi.

ARIMA Model Based analysis for West Bengal: The main sequence analysis ACF and PACF plots revealed that the series was not stationary. Modifications allowed the series transition to reach stationary. After distribution of the differentiated sequence ACF and PACF, an ARIMA model (2,2,2) was established. To validate the adequacy of the model, the Normalized Bayesian Knowledge Criterion (BIC) was tested. Again, the ARIMA (2,2,2) model was found to be the most suitable model with a Normalized BIC value of 9,914 for the recovered case model and 8,798 for the verified case model, within a class of substantially adequate ARIMA (p, d, q) models of the same dataset (Table 9.2). According to the Stationary R-squared definition, a positive R-squared means that the one to be considered is better than the reference one, which is true in this case, so we should conclude that it is a stronger one. In another observation on the Normalized Bayesian Information Criterion (BIC), it was observed that a class of statistically valid

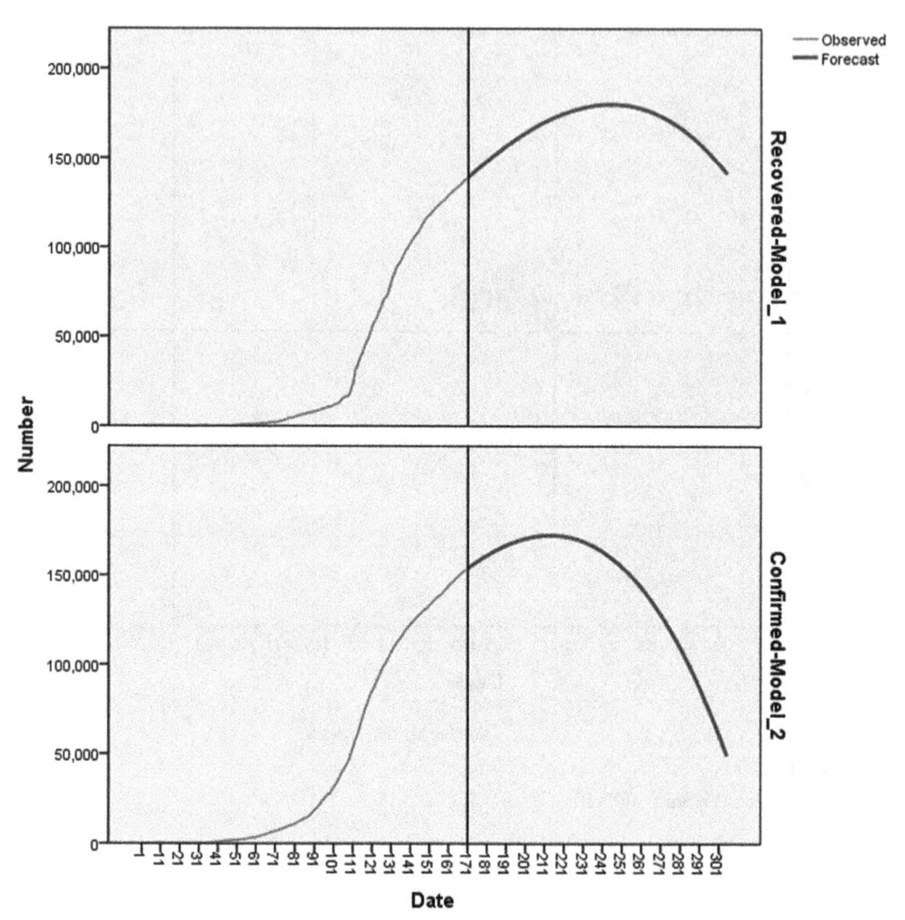

FIGURE 9.2

Forecasted Time Series for the State of Delhi.

TABLE 9.1

Time Series Modeler for the State of Delhi

Model Statistics							
Model	**Number of Predictors**	**Model Fit Statistics**		**Ljung-Box Q(18)**			**Number of Outliers**
		Stationary R-squared	**Normalized BIC**	**Statistics**	**DF**	**Sig.**	
Recovered-Model_1	1	.374	13.171	18.075	14	.203	0
Confirmed-Model_2	1	.191	11.589	43.741	14	.000	0

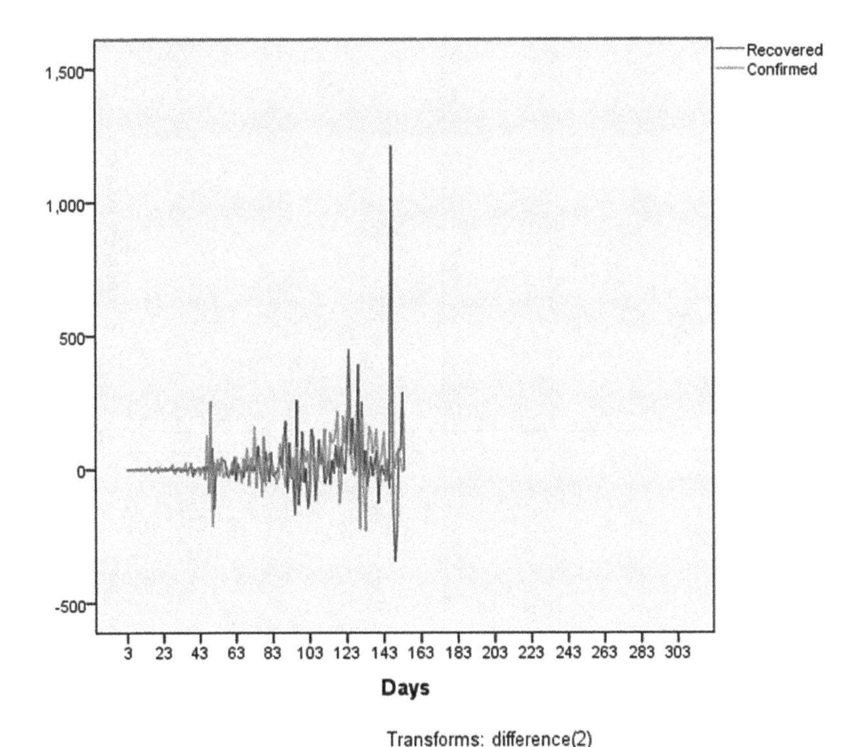

FIGURE 9.3
Sequence Plot for the State of West Bengal.

ARIMA models (p, d, q) fitted to the sequence, the ARIMA model (0,0,0) had the BIC value of 19,109 for the recovered case model, and 19,633 for the verified case model, which is far higher than our current ARIMA model (2,2,2), so we chose the new fitting model. A prediction was rendered based on the above observation as shown in Figure 9.4. The following observations were made from the forecasted data: (1) In the forecast dataset for recovered cases, the maximum number of cases will be reported in the last week of December 2020, and it could increase further. (2) In the projected dataset for confirmed cases, the largest number of cases will be reported in the last week of December 2020, and it could further increase.

ARIMA Model Based analysis for Tamil Nadu: The ACF and PACF plots of principal sequence analysis showed that the series was not stationary. Changes allowed the series transformation to stationary distance. An ARIMA model (2,2,2) was defined following distribution of the separated series ACF and PACF. To validate the adequacy of the model, the Normalized Bayesian Knowledge Criterion (BIC) was tested. Again, the ARIMA (2,2,2) model was found to be the most suitable model with a Normalized BIC value of 12,522 for the recovered case model and 10,626 for the reported case model within

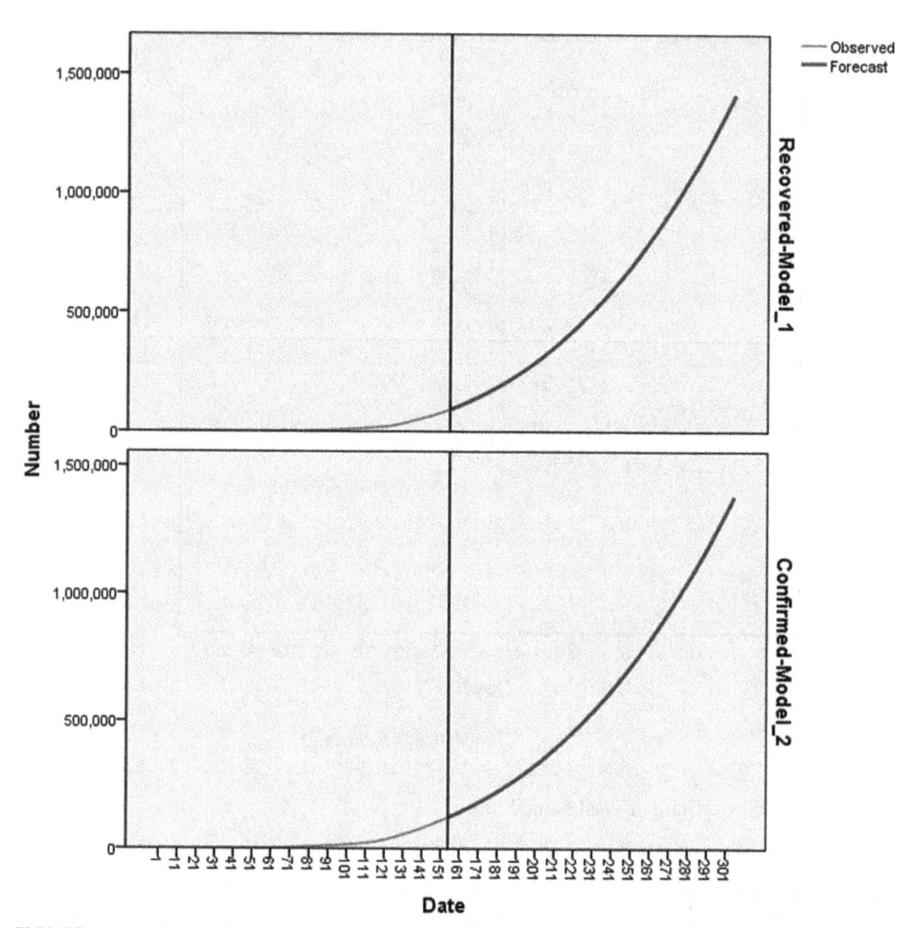

FIGURE 9.4
Forecasted Time Series for the State of West Bengal.

TABLE 9.2
Time Series Modeler for the State of West Bengal

Model Statistics							
Model	**Number of Predictors**	**Model Fit Statistics**		**Ljung-Box Q(18)**			**Number of Outliers**
		Stationary R-squared	**Normalized BIC**	**Statistics**	**DF**	**Sig.**	
Recovered-Model_1	1	.077	9.914	14.784	14	.393	0
Confirmed-Model_2	1	.076	8.798	38.074	14	.001	0

a class of substantially adequate ARIMA (p, d, q) models of the same dataset (Table 9.3). According to the Stationary R-squared definition, a positive R-squared means that the one to be considered is better than the reference one that is true in this case, so we should conclude that it is a stronger one. In another observation on the Normalized Bayesian Information Criterion (BIC), it was observed that a class of statistically valid ARIMA models (p, d, q) fitting to the sequence, the ARIMA model (0,0,0) had the BIC value of 21,474 for the retrieved case model, and 21,798 for the reported case model, which is far higher than our current ARIMA model (2,2,2) and so we choose the current one. A prediction as illustrated in Figure 9.6 was rendered based on the above observation. The following observations were made from the forecasted data: (1) In the forecast dataset for recovered cases, the maximum number of cases will be reported in the last week of December 2020, and it could increase further. (2) In the projected dataset for confirmed cases, the largest number of cases will be reported in the last week of December 2020, and it could further increase.

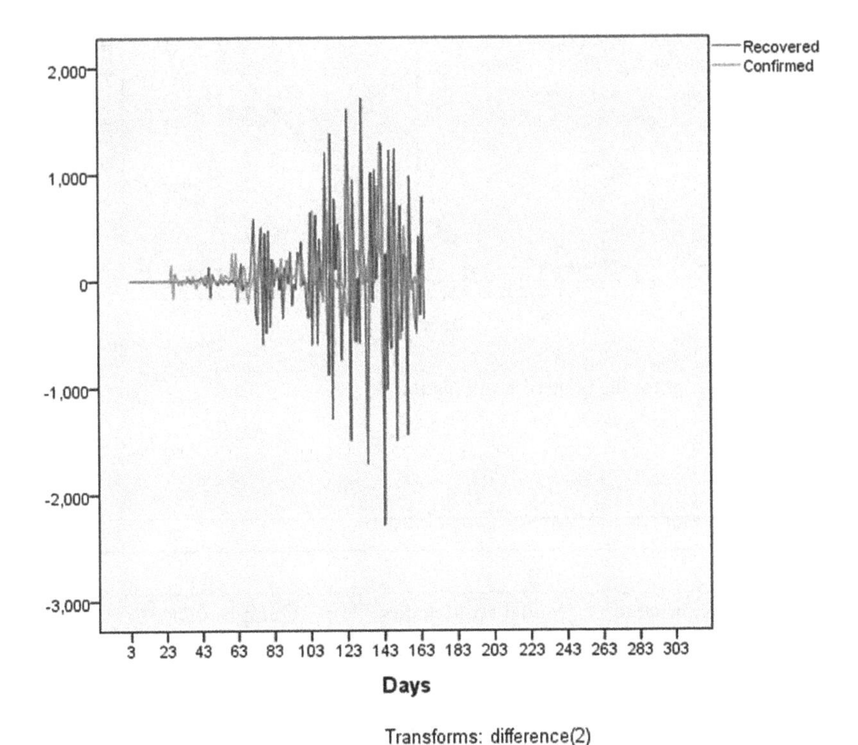

FIGURE 9.5
Sequence Plot for the State of Tamil Nadu.

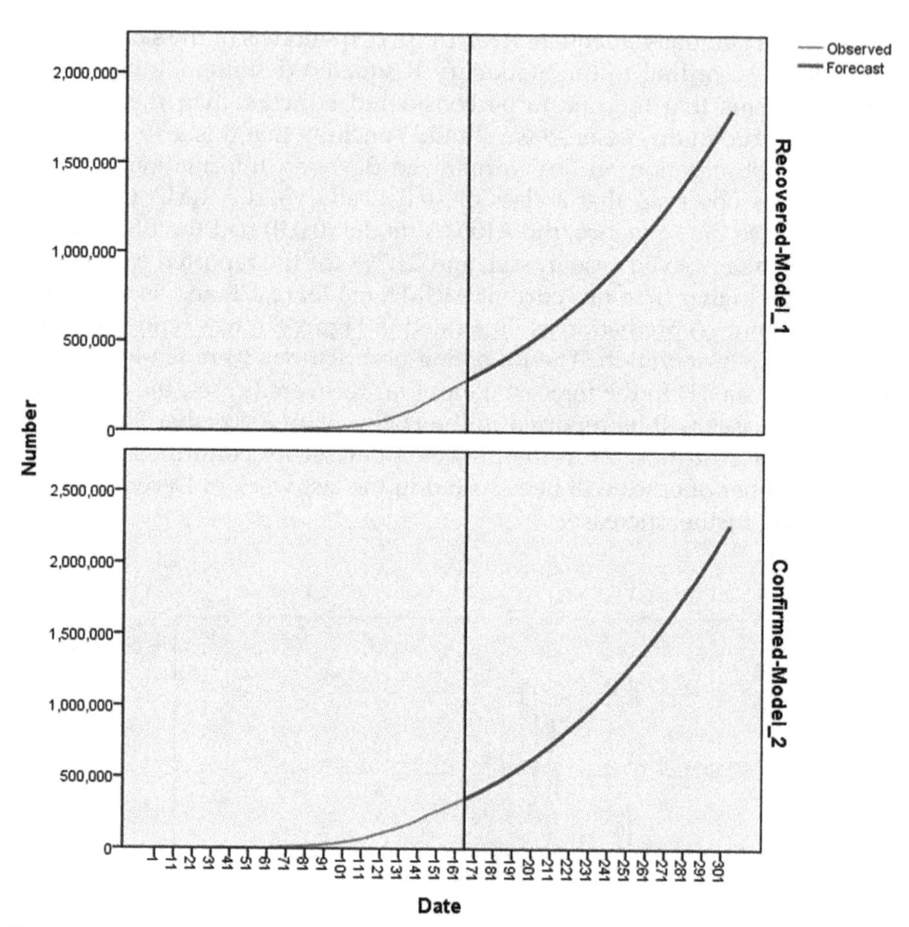

FIGURE 9.6
Forecasted Time Series for the State of Tamil Nadu.

TABLE 9.3

Time Series Modeler for the State of Tamil Nadu

Model Statistics

Model	Number of Predictors	Model Fit Statistics		Ljung-Box Q(18)			Number of Outliers
		Stationary R-squared	Normalized BIC	Statistics	DF	Sig.	
Recovered-Model_1	1	.254	12.522	24.585	14	.039	0
Confirmed-Model_2	1	.060	10.626	24.824	14	.036	0

ARIMA Model Based analysis for Maharashtra State: The main sequence analysis ACF and PACF plots revealed that the series was not stationary. Modifications allowed the series transition to reach stationary. After distribution of the differentiated sequence ACF and PACF, an ARIMA model (2,2,2) was established. To validate the adequacy of the model, the Normalized Bayesian Knowledge Criterion (BIC) was tested. Again, the ARIMA (2,2,2) model was found to be the most suitable model with a normalized BIC value of 14,453 for recovered case and 13,094 for verified case within a class of substantially adequate ARIMA (p, d, q) models of the same dataset (Table 9.4). According to the Stationary R-squared definition, a positive R-squared means that the one to be considered is better than the reference one that is true in this case, so we should conclude that it is a stronger one. In another observation on the Normalized Bayesian Information Criterion (BIC) it was observed that a class of statistically valid ARIMA models (p, d, q) fitting the sequence, the ARIMA model (0,0,0) had the BIC value of 22,084 for recovered case and 22,589 for verified case which is far higher than our current ARIMA model (2,2,2) so we can infer that the current fitting model is adequate. On the basis of the above observation a forecast as seen in Figure 9.8 was made. The following observations

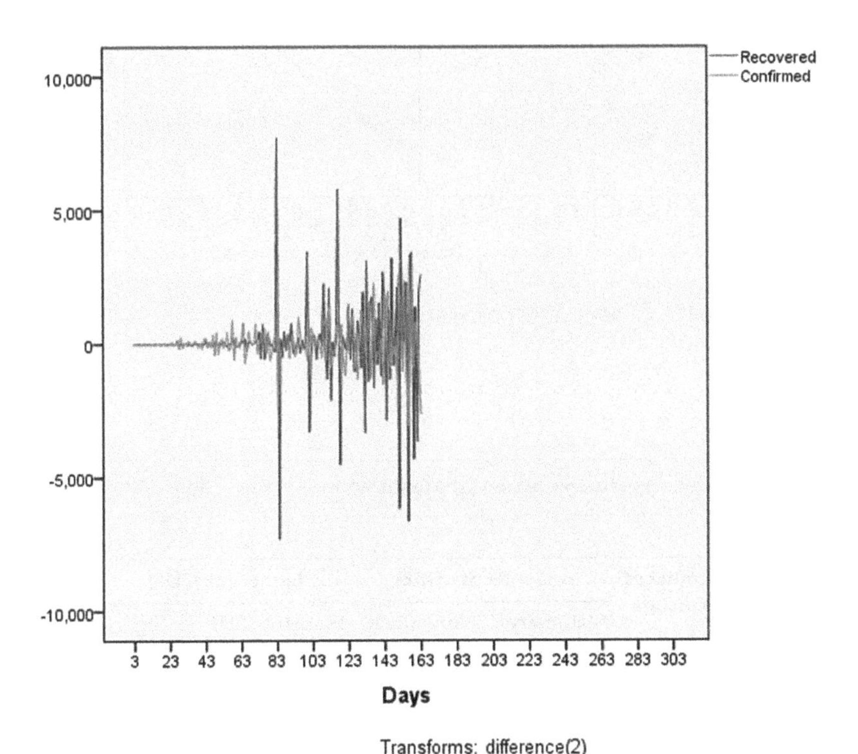

FIGURE 9.7
Sequence Plot for the State of Maharashtra.

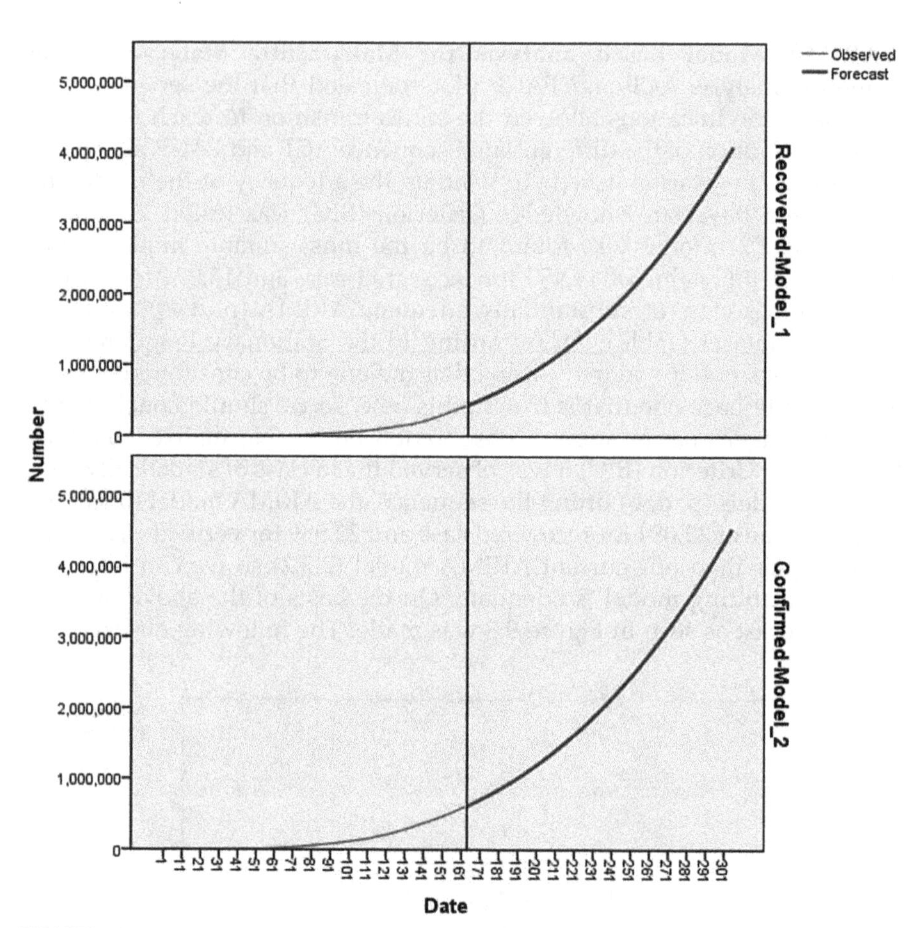

FIGURE 9.8
Forecasted Time Series for the State of Maharashtra.

TABLE 9.4
Time Series Modeler for the State of Maharashtra

Model Statistics

Model	Number of Predictors	Model Fit Statistics		Ljung-Box Q(18)			Number of Outliers
		Stationary R-squared	Normalized BIC	Statistics	DF	Sig.	
Recovered-Model_1	1	.481	14.453	27.868	14	.015	0
Confirmed-Model_2	1	.256	13.094	72.514	14	.000	0

were made from the forecasted data: (1) In the forecast dataset for recovered cases, the maximum number of cases will be reported in the last week of December 2020, and it could increase further. (2) In the projected dataset for confirmed cases, the largest number of cases will be reported in the last week of December 2020, and it could further increase.

9.5 Conclusion

The pandemic is posing a major threat for researchers as there is very limited data available during the initial stages of growth curve. The hygienic properties of the virus have not been entirely explained to date. In this chapter we have taken into consideration an upsetting major problem of the ongoing pandemic, which is successful prediction of infected cases. The procedure judges the real-time forecasting results of the daily cases in five different Indian states.

We suggested an ARIMA model that could describe the nonlinear and nonstationary behavior present in the COVID-19 cases univariate time series datasets. Forecasts for Delhi, West Bengal, Tamil Nadu and Maharashtra were given for four months ahead.

The conceptual model may be viewed as an early-alert device to counter the pandemic. We introduced a real-time forecast framework and thereby we can track the specific reported cases on a daily basis and track the forecasts. The forecasts also indicated swinging activity for the next four months and represent the effect of the state governments' broad range of social-distancing initiatives, which undoubtedly helped to contain the epidemic. Short-term forecasts do not usually indicate any strong downturn earlier. Guided by the recorded short-term predictions in this discussion, the lock-down time may be modified as needed.

References

[1] Tanujit Chakraborty & Indrajit Ghosh. Real-time forecasts and risk assessment of novel coronavirus (COVID-19) cases: A data-driven analysis. Chaos, Solitons and Fractals (2020), chaos.2020.109850.

[2] Matheus Henrique Dal Molin Ribeiro, Ramon Gomes da Silva, Viviana Cocco Mariani, & Leandro dos Santos Coelho. Short-term forecasting COVID-19 cumulative confirmed cases: Perspectives for Brazil. Chaos, Solitons and Fractals (2020), chaos.2020.109853.

[3] Domenico Benvenuto, Marta Giovanetti, Lazzaro Vassallo, Silvia Angeletti, & Massimo Ciccozzi. Application of the ARIMA model on the COVID-2019 epidemic dataset. Data in Brief, dib. 2020.105340.
[4] Nalini Chintalapudi, Gopi Battineni, & Francesco Amenta. COVID-19 virus outbreak forecasting of registered and recovered cases after sixty day lockdown in Italy: 14A data driven model approach. Journal of Microbiology, Immunology and Infection, jmii.2020.04.004.
[5] Zeynep Ceylan. Estimation of COVID-19 prevalence in Italy, Spain, and France. JScience of the Total Environment (2020), scitotenv.2020.138817.
[6] Ansari Saleh Ahmar, & Eva Boj del Val. SutteARIMA: Short-term forecasting method, a case: COVID-19 and stock market in Spain. Science of the Total Environment (2020), scitotenv.2020.138883.
[7] Hiteshi Tandon, Prabhat Ranjan, Tanmoy Chakraborty, &Vandana Suhag. Coronavirus (COVID-19): ARIMA based time-series analysis to forecast near future. Quantitative Biology, Populations and Evolution, arXiv:2004.07859.
[8] Pavan Kumar, Ram Kumar Singh, Chintan Nanda, Himangshu Kalita, Shashikanta Patairiya, Yagya Datt Sharma, Meenu Rani, & Akshaya Srikanth Bhagavathula. Forecasting COVID-19 impact in India using pandemic waves Nonlinear Growth Models. medRxiv, 2020.03.30.20047803.
[9] Rajesh Ranjan. Predictions for Covid-19 Outbreak in India Using Epidemiological Models. medRxiv, 2020.04.02.20051466.
[10] Siddique Latif, Muhammad Usman, Sanaullah Manzoor, Waleed Iqbal, Junaid Qadir, Gareth Tyson, Ignacio Castro, Adeel Razi, Maged N. Kamel Boulos, Adrian Weller, & Jon Crowcroft. Leveraging Data Science to Combat COVID-19: A Comprehensive Review. ResearchGate, 2020.
[11] Quoc-Viet Pham, Dinh C. Nguyen, Thien Huynh-The, Won-Joo Hwang, & Pubudu N. Pathirana. Artificial Intelligence (AI) and Big Data for Coronavirus (COVID-19) Pandemic: A Survey on the State-of-the-Arts. IEEE Access (Vol. 8), 130820–130839.

10

Conclusion

Rik Das, Siddhartha Bhattacharyya, and Sudarshan Nandy

Computer Aided Diagnosis (CAD) is an active area of research instrumental for identifying fatal diseases at their inception. CAD has achieved noteworthy advancements in this domain with the popularity of current disruptive trends in machine learning applications. A high level of precision superior to manual detection is observed with application of CAD systems in recognizing malignancy for terminal cancer, which has challenged the medical science for an extensive period. These systems have prevented the premature death of many patients due to late detection and several procedural formalities. Therefore, it is pertinent to design efficient algorithms for proposing CAD systems [1] to mitigate the challenges of critical illnesses at an early stage. Researchers are facing multiple challenges for preparing an automated detection system due to lack of training data, sample annotation, region of interest identification, proper segmentation and so on.

Fortunately, recent advancements in computer vision and content-based image classification have paved the way for assorted techniques to address the aforesaid challenges and have helped attain novel paradigms for designing CAD systems. Popular deep learning and machine learning application have profusely added in augmenting the detection accuracy.

This volume has made an attempt to collate novel techniques and methodologies in the domain of content-based image classification and deep learning/machine learning techniques to design efficient computer aided diagnosis architecture. It also aims to highlight new challenges and probable solutions in the domain of computer aided diagnosis to leverage a sustainable ecology.

The introductory chapter highlights the importance of computer aided diagnosis [2][3] in the present context, particularly its role in assisting early and faster detection of life-threatening diseases by minimizing the wait time for the arrival of a domain specialist to identify a particular disease. The advent of machine learning and artificial intelligence has facilitated effective diagnosis and prognosis.

The chapter also throws light on the future perspectives of computer aided diagnosis techniques for setting up a foundation for the public health sector with its assorted applications.

The contributed chapters are oriented on elucidating the basic principles of machine learning aided computer aided diagnosis with reference to several application areas, including detection of epidemics, diabetes and cardio-vascular diseases to name a few [4][5][6][7]. The chapters focuses on the challenges being encountered in today's world as far as the detection of these diseases is concerned [8]. They also put forward novel techniques for addressing these challenges, with an endnote on future extensions of the proposed techniques.

As such, the methods and techniques presented in the contributed chapters usher in a new era of intelligent computer aided diagnosis. It is strongly believed that these methods would surely benefit medical practitioners in dealing with the uncertainties involved in accurate and early detection and diagnosis of critical ailments, thereby advancing the healthcare sector and ensuring a sustainable ecological balance.

References

1. Yanase, J., & Triantaphyllou, E. (2019) A systematic survey of computer-aided diagnosis in medicine: Past and present developments. *Expert Systems with Applications*, 138: 112821.
2. Doi, K. (2007) Computer-aided diagnosis in medical imaging: historical review, current status and future potential. *Computerized medical imaging and graphics*, 31(4–5): 198–211.
3. Giger, M.L., & Suzuki, K. (2008) Computer-aided diagnosis. In *Biomedical information technology* (pp. 359–374). Academic Press.
4. Yavuz, Ü.N.A.L., & Dudak, M.N. (2020) Classification of Covid-19 dataset with some machine learning methods. *Journal of Amasya University the Institute of Sciences and Technology*, 1(1): 30–37.
5. Wang, L., & Wong, A. (2020) COVID-Net: A tailored deep convolutional neural network design for detection of COVID-19 cases from chest x-ray images. arXiv preprint arXiv: 2003.09871.
6. Zhang, J., Xie, Y., Li, Y., et al. (2020) Covid-19 screening on chest x-ray images using deep learning based anomaly detection. arXiv preprint arXiv: 2003.12338.
7. Kooi, T., Litjens, G., Ginneken, B., Gubern-Mterida, A., Stanchez, C., Mann, R., Heeten, G. & Karssemeijer, N. (2016) Large scale deep learning for computer aided detection of mammographic lesions. *Medical Image Analysis*, 35: 303–312.
8. Natalia Pirouzbakht and J. Mejia. (2017) Algorithm for the detection of breast cancer in digital mammograms using deep learning. *Proceedings of RCCS+SPIDTEC2 2017*, pp. 46–49.

Index